# BETH SHAW'S
# YOGAFIT®

### THIRD EDITION

## BETH SHAW

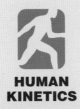

**HUMAN
KINETICS**

**Library of Congress Cataloging-in-Publication Data**

Shaw, Beth, 1966-
  [YogaFit]
  Beth Shaw's yogafit / Beth Shaw. -- Third edition.
     pages cm
  Includes bibliographical references and index.
  1.  Physical fitness. 2.  Hatha yoga.  I. Title.
  RA781.7.S446 2016
  613.7'046--dc23

                                2015020535

ISBN: 978-1-4925-0740-6 (print)

This publication is written and published to provide accurate and authoritative information relevant to the subject matter presented. It is published and sold with the understanding that the author and publisher are not engaged in rendering legal, medical, or other professional services by reason of their authorship or publication of this work. If medical or other expert assistance is required, the services of a competent professional person should be sought.

The web addresses cited in this text were current as of April 2015, unless otherwise noted.

**Acquisitions Editor:** Michelle Maloney; **Senior Managing Editor:** Amy Stahl; **Copyeditor:** Joanna Hatzopoulos Portman; **Permissions Manager:** Martha Gullo; **Senior Graphic Designer:** Nancy Rasmus; **Cover Designer:** Keith Blomberg; **Photographs (cover and interior):** David Young-Wolff, www.davidyoung-wolff.com; **Visual Production Assistant:** Joyce Brumfield; **Photo Production Manager:** Jason Allen; **Printer:** Versa Press

Human Kinetics books are available at special discounts for bulk purchase. Special editions or book excerpts can also be created to specification. For details, contact the Special Sales Manager at Human Kinetics.

Printed in the United States of America.          10   9   8   7   6   5   4   3   2

The paper in this book is certified under a sustainable forestry program.

**Human Kinetics**
Web site: www.HumanKinetics.com

*United States:* Human Kinetics
P.O. Box 5076
Champaign, IL 61825-5076
800-747-4457
e-mail: info@hkusa.com

*Canada:* Human Kinetics
475 Devonshire Road, Unit 100
Windsor, ON N8Y 2L5
800-465-7301 (in Canada only)
e-mail: info@hkcanada.com

*Europe:* Human Kinetics
107 Bradford Road
Stanningley
Leeds LS28 6AT, United Kingdom
+44 (0)113  255  5665
e-mail: hk@hkeurope.com

*Australia:* Human Kinetics
57A Price Avenue
Lower Mitcham, South Australia 5062
08 8372 0999
e-mail: info@hkaustralia.com

*New Zealand:* Human Kinetics
P.O. Box 80
Mitcham Shopping Centre, South Australia 5062
0800 222 062
e-mail: info@hknewzealand.com

# BETH SHAW'S
# YOGAFIT®

THIRD EDITION

# CONTENTS

It is an honor and a pleasure to recommend to you the third edition of Beth Shaw's wise, helpful, and constructive book titled *Beth Shaw's YogaFit, Third Edition*.

In this third edition, Beth Shaw, a woman who transplanted from New York to Los Angeles, a prodigious writer, promoter, teacher, and inspirer, has written a text that is at once accessible to those who are just beginning their yoga journey and instructive for everyone eager to advance further on that journey.

Beth has given lectures and presentations on yoga in Canada, Australia, Hong Kong, Sweden, Singapore, Turkey, Costa Rica, India, England, and Cyprus. She has taught her unique blend of yoga and fitness to many of the world's leading fitness companies including 24 Hour Fitness; Equinox; New York Sports Clubs; Spectrum; the YMCA; Gold's Gym; the International Dance and Exercise Association (IDEA); the International Health, Racquet and Sportsclub Association (IHRSA); FILEX; AsiaFit; and the Taiwanese Fitness Conference.

So, what is it about Beth Shaw's approach to yoga instruction in this book, as in so many other of her teaching venues, that puts her in such demand? I would answer that question in three ways.

First, she is a superb writer and teacher. She teaches with her text, which is always clear and never dull, and she teachers with her pictures, which are always optimally illuminative of what she is describing with her writing.

Second, and even more important, she has an obvious passion for her subject, and for how the practice of yoga—for the young as well as for the less young, and for the already adept as well as for nascent beginner—can enrich the lives of every one of us. This text is instructional, but it is also inspirational. You cannot read *Beth Shaw's YogaFit* without wanting to become more involved with yoga.

Third, and most important, this is a wise book. Beth is always supremely conscious that the people for whom she is writing are part of a broad spectrum of yoga practitioners from beginners to those who have practiced for many years. Ever so wisely, she is continually advising her readers that every body is different and every day is different so that all of us—no matter where we might be on our respective yoga journeys—need to observe and listen to what our bodies are telling us.

In this way, she operates, as it were, as a skilled and experienced physician for her thousands upon thousands of students, telling them that the real joy of yoga is the journey itself and not how much (or little) you can do on this day or that, or this year or that. I admire teachers such as Beth who, while they don't compromise on the depth and breadth of what they are teaching, they still—and at the same time—continually counsel us all that our own bodies are our most important yoga teachers.

No matter where you are on your yoga journey, read and enjoy *Beth Shaw's YogaFit, Third Edition*. It will deepen your love of and practice of yoga, at the same time moving you forward on your own unique journey.

**John McCarthy**
Executive Director Emeritus
International Health, Racquet and Sportsclub Association

YogaFit provides an easy-to-follow format for incorporating yoga into your lifestyle today. You don't need to learn Sanskrit (the original language of key yoga texts), chant, become vegetarian, do a headstand, or even be able to touch your toes to enjoy the multidimensional benefits of this ancient practice. Yoga and yoga products are everywhere in today's marketplace. People are realizing that it enhances their daily lives and generally makes them feel better; it increases range of motion in the joints and calms the mind. YogaFit is effective for everyone—active people, serious athletes, those who are sedentary, and any age group—because it is adaptable. YogaFit allows everyone to be successful in a yoga practice. Whether you are just beginning to discover the benefits of exercise or you have been working out for years, YogaFit will enrich and balance your exercise program and your ability to enjoy life. Most people discover that the more they study and practice YogaFit, the more they want to make healthier choices and alter their lifestyle to support feeling and living better.

As with any lifestyle change, slow and steady wins the race. As you read this book, take time to absorb what captures your attention. Stop and savor, just as you would during a YogaFit pose (as you will learn). Instead of rushing through the process just to get to the last chapter, stop and experience a breath or a pose that appeals to you. Observe your body and your mind even after just a few minutes of deep breathing or small, comfortable movements. Reread the book often, knowing that each time you will absorb more layers of information to bring into your practice. Embrace the idea that once the process of growth and change has begun, it will see itself through to the end. Be patient with yourself and the process.

In this book you will find many of the components of traditional yoga presented in ways that allow you to explore and adopt what you like, when you like. Yoga is not just about the physical practice of poses. It can be a way of deepening the relationship with yourself. The first part of the book focuses on the YogaFit philosophy and sets the stage for you to explore your body, mind, and spirit. **Part I,** Preparing to Be YogaFit, teaches you some of the traditional guidelines for healthier ways of interacting with yourself and the world around you as well as how workouts are structured and important breathing practices. It might be tempting to gloss over this information and skip directly to the poses, but resist doing so. These chapters come first for a reason. In order to gain the full benefits of yoga you must learn to view yoga practice through a different lens than traditional exercise. For example, yoga does not include competition; your breath sets the pace of your practice. Also, honoring your body's need for rest is just as important (and perhaps even more so) as knowing when to push. When you read and absorb part I, you will enhance your understanding of the poses and how to practice them for maximum benefit.

**Part II,** Purposeful Poses, makes up the majority of the book. The poses are classified according to general position: standing, balancing, forward bending, backward bending, and so on. Several poses have been added to the sections for this edition, and some of them may be quite challenging. Not every pose will be for every person. Also keep in mind that the journey into the pose can be exciting. Rather than getting caught up in the end result, allow yourself to have fun with exploring all dimensions of the poses. Read through all these chapters before attempting a YogaFit session, because a well-rounded workout draws from each of these chapters.

**Part III,** Putting It All Together, takes the confusion out of how to select and combine poses by offering several class formats for beginning, intermediate, and experienced practitioners. Also included are poses that complement specific sports and activities. This information allows you to feel confident starting your YogaFit journey while having the freedom to eventually create your own workouts based on your personal needs and interests.

New to this edition is the chapter titled Yoga as Therapy (chapter 11). You may be interested in yoga for healing purposes or for stress reduction, and this chapter offers poses that are more therapeutic in nature. The poses are gentle and supported, and the sessions are slower paced. Yoga can be a very effective practice for healing and re-entering activity after an injury or illness.

As my story in the introduction indicates, this book is quite literally for everybody and every *body,* with the exception of those with special or chronic conditions. As with any exercise program, before beginning your YogaFit practice, check with your doctor to ensure that this program is safe for you. What separates YogaFit from other forms of exercise is that YogaFit speaks directly and without pretentiousness to everyone, helping you and your body reach full potential.

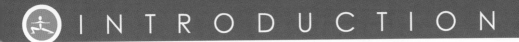

Fitness has always been a part of me. I've been working out in gyms since I was 15 years old. I enjoy few things more than moving my body in some way, be it dancing, walking my dogs, working out, or doing yoga. Wherever I am active, I feel at home. I grew up active as an avid swimmer. I would jump off my parents' boat and swim very long distances to shore, relying on yogalike breathing to stay calm and focused. As a child I also taught myself to meditate and do visualization to rid myself of horrible migraine headaches. In college I did aerobics (which I was never good at) and played some tennis. My highlight was the gym—located on the North Shore of Long Island—I went every morning as ritual. One day while stretching (yoga) I saw the sky part with a white light, and the message came to me that I would one day be very, very successful in the health and fitness industry.

After college, I moved from New York to California, where I unwittingly started a sedentary advertising sales job. I promptly gained 40 pounds. Soon after, I decided I better get things together, so I joined a gym and began going every morning at 5 o'clock. Gradually, things in my life took a turn. I swapped bean and cheese burritos for carrot sticks and hard-boiled eggs. I took control of my credit card debt and student loans. I found myself growing stronger emotionally and mentally. Exercise was literally turning my life around.

When I moved to Los Angeles, yoga was one of those seemingly "California" things I always wanted to try, like getting a waterbed and a cell phone. My first yoga teacher was Renee Taylor. After being diagnosed with cancer in the 1960s Renee had gone to live in Rishikesh, the birthplace of yoga at the basin of the Ganges River in the Himalayas. She learned the many aspects of yoga, adopted a vegetarian diet, and over time, she was healed. She came home and started teaching yoga, writing books, and making tapes. My company YogaFit now brings groups of students to Rishikesh, and I am constantly amazed by the incredible energy of the region and the effect that simply being there has on me. I have been going to India with regularity for over 7 years now.

Renee was well into her 90s when I met her. She would just sit on her desk in her carpeted studio and instruct. We did yoga on beach towels back then. I was a runner at the time, and she used to tell me, "Don't run, just do yoga." But I was initially awkward in most of my attempts. Slowly, my practice improved, and over time I mastered some poses. Visiting yoga ashrams and retreats gave me a glimpse into the more esoteric aspects of the practice. I made a whole group of yoga friends. We would attend classes and take trips together. I had found a group of like-minded people, and I look back on those days as some of my most profound. Yoga came first. I was disciplined and focused on my practice. My yoga practice led me to become a spiritual seeker. Personal growth workshops, astrology, movement expression—you name it, I did it. I looked under every rock for an answer, a spiritual experience, and a connection.

In the early 1990s, I took my first of many teacher trainings. I was soon teaching several classes a week at a variety of health clubs. It felt only right that in my teaching I would blend my love and knowledge of fitness with my yoga teachings. Students loved it! We played fun music, incorporated fitness moves, and everyone felt good. Not long after, I started producing a local cable TV yoga show called YogaFit. (The name came to me on a bike ride.)

Around that time the manager of the club approached me to turn the club's golf room into a yoga studio. In 1994 we opened what I believe was the first yoga studio within a health club in the United States. By that time I was selling my YogaFit logo wear in my classes and had really gotten the name out in the South Bay of Los Angeles. Yoga magazines were writing about my clothing and TV show, and I had produced an audiotape for an audio book company. Seeing the brand's potential, one of my yoga students, Po Chang, took a chance, invested seed money into YogaFit, and helped me incorporate. The term *angel investor* is indeed an accurate one; I could not have done any of this without his vision and support.

I opened my first YogaFit studio in early 1998. Community service was just as important to us then as it is now. We held breast cancer fundraisers, pet adoptions, and children's classes. I've always felt that no matter how big or small your business is, it is important to give back. How rich or poor you feel is relative, and we all have the power to make a positive difference on this planet in some way. To negate or ignore this natural calling and duty is to deny the essence and beauty of being a human (humane) being.

Yoga has changed my life in every possible way you can imagine, and in many ways that no one can. I am grateful for the gift of this practice daily—grateful for the opportunity to move, to breathe, to feel; grateful to be able to assist others in transformation, evolution, and awakening; grateful to be able to witness positive change in myself and others around me; grateful for the beautiful spirits that work for YogaFit and their desire to move themselves and others toward the light; grateful to have this energetic wave called YogaFit that has changed millions of lives; grateful for the opportunity to keep growing within my own yoga practice; grateful for the calling (dharma) to help animals; and grateful that YogaFit provides me the opportunity to support the animal movement in so many ways.

In his book *Growing the Positive Mind*, Dr. William K. Larkin says that the body chemistry associated with gratitude is the most optimally healthy state of mind. Research shows that a positive state of mind affects us at a cellular level. When practicing yoga, be grateful for what you can do, and the rest will come in time—when it's right, and when you are ready. The physical body is perhaps the most tangible testing ground we have. As in YogaFit's education ladder, everything starts with the physical. From there, we grow and transcend.

May we always approach our physical practice with this deep appreciation—to be in these bodies, to move, to breathe, to feel, to sweat—what a gift!

Namasté ("I bow to you")
~ **Beth Shaw**

## PART 1

# Preparing to Be YogaFit

# C H A P T E R

# YogaFit Lifestyle

Many people are curious about yoga and have heard its benefits extolled. Still, they hesitate to walk into a class for fear of not being able to touch their toes, much less bend like a pretzel. If you are one of those people, remember this fact: If you can breathe, you can do yoga. YogaFit is a user-friendly style for *every*body and every *body*. YogaFit participants are encouraged to modify and adjust poses to fit their bodies rather than the other way around. Explore this practice, and you may find out that the "secret" to touching your toes is actually bending your knees! The YogaFit Essence underlies the YogaFit philosophy and lifestyle. Become familiar with the following words and bring the essence into your yoga practice and your daily life!

YogaFit Essence:

> Breathing, feeling, listening to the body
>
> Letting go of expectations, judgments, and competition
>
> Staying in the present moment

## What Is Yoga?

Asking people to define yoga brings a variety of responses, such as balance, connection, exercise, a way to relieve stress, and more. Most people in the West are first introduced to the physical aspect of yoga, also known as hatha (pronounced *ha ta*) yoga. The Sanskrit word *hatha* means "to move by force." It is more poetically defined by looking at the root words *ha*, which means "sun," and *tha*, which means "moon." The word *yoga* means "to yoke," or to bring together all aspects of the body and mind. Hatha yoga, then, can be defined as bringing together or balancing the body and mind through a series of physical movements. The physical practice of yoga was developed to help a person sit in quiet contemplation for long periods of time, and it is just one component of the YogaFit lifestyle.

In 1994, YogaFit was born of an idea to make yoga more accessible to the Western public. In the last 20 years, YogaFit has evolved from a physical practice that introduces poses in the gym to a more holistic practice that includes teachings of the ancient yogic wisdom and lifestyle. YogaFit embraces the eight limbs (called *ashtanga* in Sanskrit) of classical Indian yoga as the way to explore the self more deeply and find deeper meaning in life. The eight limbs are as follows:

1. Yamas (restraints or ethical standards)
2. Niyamas (observances or self-regulation)
3. Asana (poses)
4. Pranayama (breathing practices)
5. Pratyahara (sense withdrawal)
6. Dharana (practicing focus on a single point)
7. Dhyana (meditation for long periods)
8. Samadhi (connection or peace)

Limbs 1 and 2 deal with the ethical practices of yoga and life, limb 3 is the physical practice, and limb 4 is the practice of breath techniques and learning to control and lengthen the breath. Limbs 5 through 7 are stair steps toward meditation. Limbs 1 to 7 are all essential in creating the peace that defines limb 8! Yoga embraces unity and diversity. Its ultimate aim is to give you a deeper connection with yourself and the world around you. For some, this aim includes a deeper connection to the Divine. Practicing one or all of these eight limbs can guide you and help you make this connection, leading to a life of greater joy, acceptance, and peace.

The practice of yoga is an inward journey that gives you a chance to cultivate awareness and health in a holistic fashion that encompasses body, mind, and spirit. Optimal health lies in taking care of all of the layers of the self. Moving inward to become more conscious of daily habits is described in yogic terms as moving through layers of consciousness, called *koshas*. Koshas (sheaths) are believed to cover the inner light of consciousness (your true beauty) beyond the physical appearance. In describing the koshas, the word *maya* (illusion) is also used. Even though many begin the practice of yoga to take care of or change their physical appearance, the yoga practice can help you move beyond the illusion that you are only a physical being. Like washing mud off of the headlights of a car, you begin to gain a clearer picture of the truth of your life journey and a deeper spiritual connection.

The outermost layer is the physical body (called *annamaya kosha*), which you nourish with food and exercise. The next layer is the energy body (called *pranamaya kosha*); the yoga practice can help you become aware of how and where your energy flows and how you can maximize positive energy flow. The third layer is the mental or emotional (called *manomaya kosha*), where awareness of your emotional and mental state can help you lessen anxiety and other moods that negatively affect your health. The YogaFit lifestyle guides you toward acceptance and understanding of the interplay of your emotions and your reactions. The fourth layer is referred to as the wisdom layer (called *vijnanamaya kosha*). This wisdom is cultivated with your practice, and it helps you realize what is useful and what to let go of. The fifth layer is known as the bliss layer (*anandamaya kosha*). The fifth layer can be described as true peace or inner happiness that isn't reliant on anything external but instead just being. There is nothing you can do to disturb the bliss layer. It is simply a matter of discovering what is already there. The first four layers are affected by your daily thoughts, words, and actions; they interact and affect the other layers like ripples in a pond. For example, if you have pain in the physical body, tension develops, movement and thinking patterns change, and consequently energy flow is interrupted. Pain anywhere in the body tends to bring up emotions that could keep you in a negative thinking pattern. As you increase your awareness, you realize you have a choice in how you live your life and that each choice you make has an effect on your whole self and on those around you. Only when you can bring the unconscious into the light of awareness can you begin to find happiness and true freedom. This consciousness and attention to presence is the true gift of the yoga practice.

The YogaFit lifestyle is having the gift of freedom in your body, mind, and spirit, and living a pain-free life in every respect. The YogaFit lifestyle is also about creating space both physically and mentally. In that space lies more freedom. Yoga differs from a traditional exercise regimen because of the mindful aspect of the practice. Yoga asks you to pay attention not only to the body but also to your thoughts, words, and actions, both on and off the mat. This attention increases awareness and sets the stage for transformation. Truly embracing the YogaFit lifestyle is a step toward creating optimal health of the body and mind.

In the Western world most people doing yoga are practicing the physical component of yoga known as *hatha yoga*. All physical yoga is hatha yoga. For many, the practice of yoga postures, called asanas, creates a desire to embrace the entire spectrum that is yoga. The YogaFit essence, the four paths of yoga, and the foundation of yoga philosophy—the eight limbs (ashtanga) of classical Indian yoga (described previously)—are the springboards for taking your yoga practice off your mat. Whether you choose to focus on asana (postures) and pranayama (breathing practices) or meditation, or you choose to study the other various aspects of yoga as well, ultimately you will enhance your personal awareness and understanding beyond your physical body.

YogaFit vinyasa yoga is part of the ongoing evolution of yoga in the West. The word *vinyasa* means literally "to place in a special way," but it is also commonly called "flow" yoga, because you move fluidly with the breath from one pose to the next. Linking the poses in this way creates strength, flexibility, endurance, and balance for greater health and mental awareness. YogaFit vinyasa yoga complements other styles of yoga. It has a familiar focus to other styles, yet it also includes stylistic elements that make it unique.

Remember that everyone's yoga journey is different; feel free to pursue your yoga practice to the degree that is comfortable for you.

# YogaFit Essence

The essence of the YogaFit lifestyle is breathing, feeling, and listening to your body; letting go of expectation, judgment, and competition; and staying in the present moment.

The foundation for a successful YogaFit lifestyle is in your ability to practice the essence of YogaFit both on and off the mat. As you read the following elements of the YogaFit essence, consider where you might apply them to your daily life. Then, once you begin practicing the poses and workout formats, notice how they enhance your experience in the poses.

• **Breathing.** Breathing is vitally important to your yoga practice because it gives you energy, keeps you in the moment, and facilitates the process of unifying mind, body, and spirit. Breathing during your YogaFit session is typically done through the nose. Deep diaphragmatic breathing is the key to a successful asana and meditation practice. The breath is your most powerful tool for calming and relaxing your body and clearing your mind; in fact, if you are not ready to begin a physical practice, just doing 5 to 10 minutes a day of deep diaphragmatic breathing will begin to bring you the positive health benefits of yoga. Effective breathing also helps you get deeper into your poses. Regardless of the pose, you should always focus on maintaining a long, smooth breath. (See chapter 3 for details on YogaFit breathing techniques.)

• **Feeling and listening to your body.** In the Western world people are often disconnected from their physical bodies. Yoga can help reconnect the body, mind, and spirit. You should aim to feel something in every pose. During practice, remind yourself to check in with your body and to modify your pose to provide less or more sensation, as appropriate. When you feel something in each pose, you are grounded in the moment and aware of your body and its potential. The ability to identify and feel your feelings gives you tremendous opportunity to connect with yourself and with others honestly.

• **Letting go of expectations.** Too often in life people have unrealistic expectations of themselves and others. These expectations can manifest in your yoga practice and lead to injury on the mat. Be patient with your practice. Respect the process, and go at your own pace.

• **Letting go of competition.** As the great yoga philosopher J. Krishnamurti said, when you compare, you are disappointed. Your practice is your own. No two bodies are alike, and no two lives are alike. Comparison makes you feel either superior or inferior. Neither is beneficial.

- **Letting go of judgment.** It is no one's place to judge others' lifestyles or actions. Practice replacing judgment with compassion. Do you want to be judged by others for the way you look or for the way you are? Think of how unfairly you feel treated when someone who barely knows you misjudges you. The truth is that most judgments are based on inadequate information. Ask yourself how much you know about a person you have placed a judgment on. Ask yourself why you feel compelled to make a judgment. Is it to make yourself feel better? Taking it one step further, when you notice yourself judging another person, you can simply turn the mirror toward yourself. It is a tough practice, but everyone needs to remember that you cannot notice anything in others that isn't present in yourself. This step can then give you a chance to practice compassion for yourself and for others.

- **Staying in the present moment.** In his book *The Power of Now* (2004), Ekhart Tolle argues that true peace can be found only in the present moment. Tolle says that the present moment is the only moment in which you can truly live your life. When you're stuck in the past or projecting into the future, you miss out on what's in front of you. On your mat, notice when your mind slips into thoughts of the past or future. If it does, simply bring your awareness back to your breath and your body.

## Philosophy of Yoga

Yoga is a path with a rich philosophy, and the path is open to everyone. Integral to this philosophy are the first two limbs of the eight-limbed path, the yamas and niyamas, which make up 10 guidelines for leading a happier, healthier, and more conscious life. These guidelines are discussed later in this chapter. The third limb, asana, is addressed throughout this book. Chapters 3 and 12 contain more information on limbs 4 through 7 (pranayama, pratyahara, dharana, and dhyana), which are essential for meditation. The eighth limb, samadhi (peace, connection), can't be practiced or taught but is reached through practice of limbs 1 to 7. Many people look to the yamas and niyamas as a simple and appropriate way to live their lives in today's world. In times of stress or conflict, they are powerful tools to help you maintain

As my yoga practice progressed, I noticed that I naturally desired a deeper level of understanding of the various aspects that comprise yoga. I became the witness to myself, to my actions, and to the ripple effect every action created. I started to desire less—less clutter, food, stimulants and depressants, possessions, mental chatter, drama, confusion, and empty conversation. I craved more peace and calm— more harmony, tranquility, simplicity, natural beauty, truth, and space. Now when faced with a conflict, crisis, challenge, decision, or fork in the road, I refer to the yamas and niyamas to help guide and inspire me.

balance and connection with a power greater than yourself. You can think of them as nonjudgmental guideposts along the journey of life, giving you principles to guide your thoughts, words and actions.

## Yamas

The yamas are guidelines for how people interact with each other and the outer world. They are social disciplines to guide you in your relationships with others. The yamas are ahimsa (nonviolence), satya (truthfulness), asteya (nonstealing), brahmacharya (moderation), and aparigraha (noncoveting or nonattachment).

### Ahimsa (Nonviolence)

Ahimsa is the practice of nonviolence toward yourself and other living beings in your actions, thoughts, and speech. Not only do you cause no harm, you do not accept or allow anything that causes harm. Because violence arises out of fear, anger, restlessness, and selfishness, ahimsa advocates kindness, compassion, love, patience, self-love, and worthiness. Ahimsa must start with the self and is based on the reality that everything is connected. If you treat yourself poorly, then you cause harm to yourself and to those around you. The reverse is true as well. Ahimsa is considered to be the foundation of yoga and is woven through all the other yamas and niyamas.

*YogaFit essence:* Listen to your body and even your inner dialogue (self-talk) to help you in your yoga practice. Practice with a sense of self-acceptance and love for exactly where you are in your practice today.

### Satya (Truthfulness)

Satya is truthfulness in speech, thoughts, and deeds. To practice satya is to exhibit honesty (with the intention of helping, not harming) while owning your feelings, valuing genuine and gentle communication, giving constructive feedback, forgiving and letting go of judgment, and taking off your "mask."

*YogaFit essence:* Go at your own pace; be honest about what that pace is. When moving into a pose, notice if you are trying to move in your own true range of motion. Rather than make your body fit the pose, you can make the pose fit your body.

### Asteya (Nonstealing)

Asteya embodies taking only what belongs to you. The guidelines for asteya include not stealing, not taking more than you need, including the earth's natural resources, and not being jealous. Practice asteya by using objects the right way, managing your time, cultivating a sense of completeness and self-sufficiency, and letting go of your cravings. Being mindful of how much water you use, how much food you eat, and even the type of diet that you consume is practicing asteya.

*YogaFit essence:* Let go of competition and judgment. When you stop comparing, you let go of jealousy. Letting go of expectations or the attitude of "right to have" helps you consider the well-being of others as well as your own well-being.

### Brahmacharya (Moderation)

Brahmacharya is moderation in all things on all levels. The guidelines for brahmacharya include channeling your emotions; practicing self-containment; not overindulging your mind, speech, or body; and tempering your use of sex, food, and all aspects of daily life, including the environment. To practice brahmacharya is to be mindful of how you use your energy and not to be repressed but rather to control sensual cravings.

*YogaFit essence:* Feel and listen to your body. When you're truly connected you'll rarely overindulge.

### Aparigraha (Nonattachment)

Aparigraha is letting go of reliance on possessions and relationships (attachments) for your peace and happiness. When you let go of your "stuff" and your "baggage," you face yourself. Letting go is not always comfortable, but it is always invigorating. Attachments can also be to food, jobs, even identities. These things in and of themselves aren't bad, but if you rely too much on your attachments then you stifle your room for growth. To practice aparigraha is to simplify—to distinguish needs from wants, to consume less and live more.

*YogaFit essence:* Let go of expectations. When you refrain from excess expectations, you no longer desire to fill yourself with ultimately unfulfilling possessions, addictions, and distractions.

The yoga practice should teach compassion, love, acceptance, and a desire to honor all living creatures.

## Niyamas

The niyamas are guidelines for how you interact with yourself and your internal world. The practice of the niyamas harnesses the energy generated from your practice and cultivation of the yamas. Niyamas are about self-regulation, helping you maintain a positive environment in which to grow. The five niyamas are shaucha (cleanliness), santosha (equanimity or contentment), tapas (internal fire or discipline), swadhyaya (self-observation), and ishwara-pranidhana (surrender).

### Shaucha (Cleanliness)

Shaucha is external as well as internal purity. To practice shaucha is to clear your mind and body of toxins and negative energy; to exhibit evenness of mind, thoughts, and speech; and to practice discrimination. You do this through good health habits, including eating a clean, organic diet, living in a clear and orderly environment, using cruelty-free products, and refraining from excessive amounts of stimulants and depressants, including prescription drugs, coffee, alcohol, and processed foods.

*YogaFit essence:* When you practice yogic breathing (pranayama), you cleanse your body and mind of toxins.

### Santosha (Equanimity)

Santosha invites you to maintain equanimity (evenness of mind) through all that life offers. The guidelines for santosha include contentment, accepting what is, and making the best out of everything. To practice santosha is to exhibit gratitude and joyfulness, remain calm with success or failure, let go of attachment to any external status, remain focused in the face of adversity, and choose love over fear. In *The Power of Now*, Ekhart Tolle (2004) explains that when faced with a challenging situation you can choose removal, change, or acceptance. You get to decide how to find contentment.

*YogaFit essence:* Be present in the moment, accepting with contentment that which you are immersed in at any given moment. Live in a state of flow.

### Tapas (Internal Fire)

The word *tapas* means "heat" or "fire" and is the practice of both mental and physical discipline. The guidelines for tapas are austerity, sacrifice, and enthusiasm for the spiritual path—regardless of how difficult—and a willingness to do what is necessary in order to reach a goal with discipline. To practice tapas is to exhibit determination in pursuing daily practices and your life's mission, while remaining joyful in the knowledge that outer discipline will lead to inner discipline. Tapas reminds you that obstacles are part of the path and to stay the course through difficult circumstances.

*YogaFit essence:* Stay in the present moment regardless how uncomfortable it becomes. Go through the heat and accept it, inviting it in; the fire brings transformation.

### Swadhyaya (Self-Observation)

Swadhyaya is the practice of self-observation. It gives you a pause between stimulus and response, giving you room to breathe, relax, feel, watch, and allow. Matters you are pondering might become clear to you in an almost organic manner, or it might take time for truth to emerge. Be open and cultivate the spirit of exploration within you. The guidelines of swadhyaya are self-education and study. To practice swadhyaya is not to become self-absorbed but to exhibit reflection, meditation, and a desire to know the truth.

*YogaFit essence:* Let go of expectations of yourself to allow yourself to observe speech, thoughts, and actions honestly, without judgment. This practice leads to acceptance, which leads to growth.

### *Ishwara-Pranidhana (Surrender)*

The guidelines of ishwara-pranidhana are surrendering to God, to another higher power, or to the light and energy of the universe. To practice ishwara-pranidhana is to exhibit faith, dedication, sincerity, and patience to transcend the ego, which is resistant to surrender. Ishwara-pranidhana is about your relationship to the divine energy of the universe. Your divine relationship might manifest in many ways, such as chanting, painting, being in nature or with animals, listening to music, or writing a poem. Everyone has a way to surrender to spirit and celebrate the universal connection.

*YogaFit essence:* When you let go of judgment, you let go of trying to control. Only then can you overcome your ego and celebrate connection to that which is beyond you.

# Four Paths of Yoga

Practicing the YogaFit essence and the yamas and niyamas can guide you in living a yogic life both on and off your mat, but many people also choose to deepen their practice and foster growth by following one or more of the four yoga paths. While your unique personality will dictate which paths you are most inclined to pursue on your journey, all paths lead to greater wisdom, connection and, eventually, the ability to surrender. The four paths are karma yoga, jnana yoga, raja yoga, and bhakti yoga.

1. **Karma yoga:** Selfless service

   Karma yoga is the realization of the Divine through works and duty. Karma yoga is also the basis for YogaFit's mission. This is the path of selfless service and giving. Practice karma yoga by giving back wherever you feel called, whether it's caring for friends and family, volunteering for charities and other service work, or as a YogaFit instructor teaching community service classes. When Master Vivekananda brought yoga to the United States in 1891, he said that karma yoga is the most important yoga you can do; YogaFit agrees. Since its first teacher trainings in 1997, YogaFit has had a community service program.

2. **Jnana yoga:** Knowledge

   Jnana yoga is the realization of the Divine through the acquisition of knowledge. It is the path of pursuing wisdom and intellect. Those who prefer to seek understanding through studying the words and wisdom of others are drawn to this path. If you love to study, find the texts and teachers that speak to your heart.

3. **Raja yoga:** Meditation

   Raja yoga is the realization of the Divine through control of the mind and the practice of listening. This is the path of meditation. Because the yoga postures were originally created to help you quiet your mind and body for meditation, hatha yoga is included in this path. This path is the eight limbs that ready the mind and body to sit in meditation. For many people, the answers to their questions come only through practicing stillness.

4. **Bhakti yoga:** Devotion

Bhakti yoga is the realization of the Divine through a devotion to and love of a personal God. It is the path of love and worship. Regardless of where and how you choose to worship, practicing bhakti yoga involves focusing your heart and your efforts on the Divine.

Remember that no one path is better than another. Ultimately, they all lead to that place of ishwara-pranidhana (surrender).

# Your Path

How you interpret these elements of yoga practice is subjective, and they often change as you grow. Yoga is not a religion, nor is it intended to conflict with anyone's culture or belief system. Rather, yoga is a way to dissolve barriers and engender a deeper connection between yourself and others, and between yourself and the universal spirit.

So, take what you like and leave the rest. For these concepts to have a positive impact on your life, you must be prepared to hear the truth that is spoken to your heart and to apply it. It takes work (tapas) to live your truth, but the rewards are immediate. YogaFit is a workout, yes, but it is so much more. A fit body certainly improves your quality of life and helps you live your life with vitality instead of being a prisoner to your body. However, true peace and joy are found when the body, mind, and spirit are strong and healthy. The eight limbs of yoga address the body, mind, and spirit and how to take care of them. The YogaFit lifestyle can set you free of expectations and judgment, allowing you to be free to express your true nature. Be patient with yourself during the process. Growth takes time, but once it has begun, it never stops. Embrace your journey.

# YogaFit Essentials

 Welcome to your yoga journey. Now that you understand the YogaFit lifestyle, it's time to begin your practice. One of the beautiful things about yoga is that you can do it just about anywhere and anytime. You can be indoors or outdoors; you can take it with you when you travel; and you can do it in the office or on a plane, boat, or train. This book discusses ways to incorporate YogaFit into your life. The YogaFit program has become a way of life for many people, transforming millions of lives. In this chapter, you will find out how.

## Benefits of YogaFit

A regular YogaFit workout gives you all the benefits of a traditional yoga practice and more. To achieve the best fitness results, practice three to five times a week for 30 to 60 minutes per workout. If you are coming to yoga for stress reduction, then consider a daily practice for as little as 10 to 20 minutes a session. Lavretsky et al. (2013) revealed shorter, more frequent practice may be best for reducing anxiety and stress and easier to fit into your busy schedule. Most people can probably find 10 minutes to carve out of their day to come to their mats and breathe and move. If you are new to exercise or have trouble sticking to an exercise program, starting with a daily short practice can help you create a positive daily habit that is enjoyable so that you are more likely to keep at it. The important thing is that you start your practice. You will notice the benefits quickly, which will motivate you to perhaps increase the length and the intensity when you are ready. The more you practice YogaFit, the more benefits you receive, although most people experience a positive difference after just one workout. The benefits of a mindful YogaFit practice are many and include the following:

- Increased flexibility
- Stronger muscles
- Better body tone
- A naturally defined physique
- A relaxed and clear mind
- Reduced stress
- Increased body awareness
- Natural weight loss
- Improved posture
- A strengthened immune system
- Decreased physical effects of aging for the brain and body

In recent years, yoga researchers have confirmed many of the benefits of yoga touted in the ancient texts. In addition, exciting research in the last few years has shown yoga practitioners to have stronger immune systems; changes in gene expression leading to healthier and longer lives; and decreases in anxiety, stress, and depression. A study in 2012 at the University of Illinois compared doing 20 minutes of yoga to doing aerobic exercise for the same amount of time. Researchers found that students were better able to focus and had faster reaction times after the yoga compared to traditional aerobic exercise (Gothe et al. 2013). Another study compared walking with yoga. The results showed that the yoga group had better improvements in mood, lower anxiety scores, coupled with increased levels of a mood-improving neurotransmitter called gamma-aminobutyric acid (GABA) (Streeter et al. 2010). A study funded by the NIH and published in the journal *Cerebral Cortex* in 2013 found that yoga practitioners had a higher amount of gray matter in the brain region that processed pain, as well the area that integrated body sensations. The amount of increase in gray matter correlated positively with the time in which a person practiced yoga. The yoga practitioners tolerated pain better than nonpractitioners, and the researchers said the results pointed to a difference in cognitive processing as a result of the yoga (Villemure et al. 2013). Telomeres are the ends of DNA, and the wearing out and shortening of telomeres are linked with aging and disease (Epel et al. 2006). A relatively new area of research has been showing that mindfulness meditation and yoga have a positive influence on telomeres. A recent study looking at survivors of breast cancer showed an increase in telomerase, an enzyme that protects the ends of the telomeres, with mindfulness-based meditation and group support (Carlson et al. 2015). Mindfulness meditation is maintaining an awareness of the present by focusing on something such as the breath, as is done in the YogaFit practice. Along with the benefits of a traditional yoga practice, a regular YogaFit workout also helps you succeed in your athletic endeavors by reducing the risk of injury through a greater mind–body connection; creating a more effective metabolic exchange during physical activity through better breathing patterns; offsetting the unevenness of other exercise programs by offering a complete and balanced mind–body workout for all muscle groups; and increasing endurance, willpower, and discipline by working both your body and your mind. (See chapter 10 for details on using YogaFit to cross-train with your favorite sports.)

# Preparing for Your YogaFit Workout

To prepare for your workout, create an optimal atmosphere for your yoga experience.

### Practice with the body you have today.

Approach your yoga practice with the body that you have today, not the body you had 10 years ago or even last month. Your body is different every day, so be aware of your body's needs and requirements before, during, and after your YogaFit session. Over time you'll learn what's best for your body at any given moment. Until then, relax, and try to listen to your body at all times. One of the main benefits of yoga is that you learn to *listen* to your body.

- **Know your limits.** Consider reading this entire book before you jump into your YogaFit program. For ultimate success and safety, before your first workout you should read at least all of part I (which presents balanced workout formats) and the descriptions of any poses in part II that you want to try. Before starting this program or any other new workout, check with your physician, especially if you have injuries, special conditions, or chronic illnesses or if you are pregnant, over 65, or not currently participating in a regular exercise program. Also see the section titled Special Considerations for YogaFit at the end of this chapter for ideas on how to modify your workout in accordance with your condition.

- **Take your time.** Reread sections of this book until you absorb all that YogaFit has to offer. Don't rush. You'll benefit most by going slowly through your first session at your own pace. Stop for breaks when you need them.

- **Allow time for meals and snacks to digest.** Before beginning your YogaFit session, allow at least 90 minutes after a meal so that your body has time to digest. If you think you need a snack during that 90 minutes, choose fruit, tea, or a protein drink. Just make sure you consume it at least 30 minutes before you begin your practice.

- **Give yourself space; stop all other activity at least 15 minutes before each practice.** Use the time before your session to calm, collect, and center yourself. This is a good time to prepare your practice space. Turn off (or tone down) harsh lighting. Light candles and play music to create an atmosphere that helps you focus. Leave your everyday thoughts behind, as discussed later in this chapter.

- **Position in an open space that is away from mirrors.** Roll out your mat with enough space to allow room for your arms and legs to move freely.

Avoid being too close to walls, doors, or furniture. Don't face mirrors, because they draw your focus away from how your body feels. (You'll focus on how you look instead.) Relax your face into a natural smile. Consciously release any holding patterns in your face, neck, and shoulders. Make adjustments that seem right to you. Your YogaFit session should be an enjoyable experience that you want to return to.

• **Maintain a positive mental attitude.** For success with your YogaFit session, begin with an open mind. The practice of yoga is a fluid one, a life-long journey of change and transformation. Your practice might change from one day to the next, but maintain faith in the process. As with any exercise program, you will see and feel results over time. A positive attitude is an important part of your practice because your thoughts directly influence your body chemistry and immune system. What you think determines whether you are working for your body or against it.

• **Know your range of motion and flexibility.** Everyone wants to be as strong and flexible as bamboo, but each body is different in type, flexibility, and fitness level. Therefore, two people looking alike in the same pose is not likely. A "perfect fit" varies from person to person. This variety is an aspect of yoga that keeps things interesting. You're always trying to learn what works best for your own body. No two bodies respond to the same stretch in exactly the same way. Never force, push, or shove yourself into a pose. Instead, use breathing techniques (see chapter 3) to enhance your practice.

Whether or not you have an unusually limited range of motion, focusing on proper alignment and breathing rather than on achieving maximum flexibility will lead to a safe practice. Feeling and listening to your body will help you decide when to choose modifications of various poses (see part II) in order to work muscle groups without strain or risk of injury.

Remember that you should make the pose fit your body rather than make your body fit the pose.

# What You Need to Begin YogaFit

This section discusses what you need in order to begin your program. For more information on many of the products discussed in this section, refer to appendix B.

## Clothing

Wear comfortable and snug but nonbinding clothing. You'll be sweating and stretching when you practice, and your skin tends to absorb what's next to it, so consider clothing made from organic bamboo or organic cotton. Shirts that are too loose will ride up during certain poses, so women often prefer tank tops with built-in sports bras, tights, flex pants, or capris. Men wear shorts, tank tops, or long-sleeve T-shirts. Layering is a good idea because you'll warm up and cool down. And don't forget: no shoes, no socks. YogaFit is best done barefoot.

## Yoga Mat

Many yoga mats on the market have slick surfaces that quickly deteriorate. To ensure you get a high-quality mat with staying power, buy from a vendor that specializes in yoga accessories. Because your body will often be in direct contact with your mat, consider an eco-friendly or organic mat. These mats are also better for the environment.

You can decide for yourself whether you want a thin mat or a thick mat. Some prefer thin mats because they're almost like practicing directly on the floor surface, allowing for maximum stability. But thick mats provide extra cushioning and often are best for people with knee discomfort on hard floors.

## Hard Surface

For your YogaFit session, place your mat on a wooden floor or another hard, flat, and smooth surface. Use a firm foundation that offers balance and provides optimal alignment for your joints.

## Props

Props include YogaFit egg blocks, straps, chairs, rolled-up yoga mats or blankets, and even walls. Without props, many people can't get the full benefits of the YogaFit poses. Props aren't necessarily intended to make poses easier; rather, they allow you to find a position that you can hold longer without overstretching or straining so you can focus on increasing strength and flexibility. Props can also help you overcome hesitancy and find balance, thereby boosting your confidence and promoting a feeling of success—without which you might not return to your mat.

The props listed here can make the YogaFit poses safe and effective for everyone, no matter your body type. See appendix B for details on where to purchase these items.

- **YogaFit egg blocks.** YogaFit egg blocks are lightweight foam in the shape of eggs in order to contour to the shape of the back. (See Purpose of Using Props in chapter 11.) They can also be used in poses in which tightness or unsteadiness prevents you from reaching the floor without overstretching or coming out of alignment. In these poses, you place one or both hands on the egg block. They are also great for restorative yoga as you can really relax and surrender with them supporting you. Because the gentle rounded shape of the eggs contour to the body without feeling the hard edge of a traditional block, you are able to relax a little more fully in many of the poses supported by the egg blocks.

- **Straps.** Yoga straps are useful for people with limited flexibility or injury concerns. Straps allow you to practice a pose that might otherwise be impossible or difficult, allowing you to realize the benefits of the pose with comfort. The pose chapters indicate when a strap might be helpful to modify a pose. If you don't own a strap, use a bathrobe belt or a necktie.

- **Chair.** A chair is useful for added height for forward movements, for balance, and for simple inversions.

# YogaFit's Seven Principles of Alignment

In YogaFit, yoga postures are expressed in terms of seven principles of alignment (SPA). These principles help create the optimal biomechanical positioning for your body during movement and while you're holding your YogaFit poses. The SPA increase safety while providing functional mechanical principles that you can apply in your daily life. Following is a brief explanation for each of the seven principles.

1. **Establish a base and dynamic tension.**

   For maximum stability, mobility, and extension, build your poses from the ground up by establishing a firm foundation. If your hands are on the mat, spread your fingers wide. If your feet are on the mat, distribute your weight evenly across your feet and press down to form a strong base. Next, stack your joints. For example, if you're on all fours, align your shoulders over your wrists and your hips over your knees. This alignment allows you to build strength in and protect your joints from injury. Finally, contract your muscles and extend outward through your limbs and the crown of your head. This contraction and directional energy create dynamic tension, which increases your energy and effectiveness in every pose. For example, in warrior II (see part II) you reach out in opposite directions through your fingers while reaching up through the crown of your head and sinking into the lunge.

2. **Create core stability.**

   The muscles of your midsection (abdominals, lower back, gluteal muscles, hip flexors) make up your core. Engage these muscles before moving into poses and while holding poses to create strength, stability, and mobility. You started creating your core stability when you found your base. Using the same warrior II as earlier, pressing the four corners of your feet into the mat and then lifting through arches as if you are drawing the energy up through the feet and legs and into the torso (core) to create the dynamic tension, you may notice your core already beginning to activate. When you work from a stable core, you can move with confidence into your poses and hold them with greater ease.

3. **Align the spine.**

   The spine is supported through core stabilization. When moving into twists, side bends, forward bends, or backward bends, always start by engaging your core and finding your neutral spine. (Be as tall as you can while keeping the natural curves in your spine.) This engagement strengthens your muscles in proper alignment and helps prevent injury. Remember that the head and neck are part of the spine and always follow the movement of the spine. Aligning the spine builds strength in alignment and prevents tension from increasing in your neck and shoulders.

4. **Soften and align the knees.**

   In any standing pose in which one or both of the legs are straight, keep a soft bend in the knee (or knees) to avoid locking out the joint(s). In YogaFit, this soft bend is termed a *microbend*. The microbend helps stabilize and protect the joint by strengthening surrounding muscles and corrects any muscular imbalances in the legs. Refer to poses such as warrior I, kneeling or crescent lunge, and chair, in which you stack your knees above your ankles and point them directly over your toes. In general, the knees, when bent, remain in the same line as the hips.

5. **Relax the shoulders back and down.**

   When stressed, fatigued, or tense, your shoulders tend to rise up toward your ears, which increases tension in your upper body and decreases core stability. So, in any pose, even those with arms overhead such as in warrior I (see part II), or with hands on the mat as in downward-facing dog (see part II), slide your shoulder blades toward your hip pockets and draw the tips of your shoulder blades toward your spine to open your chest.

6. **Hinge at the hips.**

   When moving into and out of forward bends, bend your knees and hinge at your hips, using the natural pulley system of your hip joints. This action will allow you to maintain a neutral spine and prevent injuries to your lower back. Come out of forward bends the same way, bending your knees a lot, finding neutral spine, then using the legs to return to a standing position. Also use this movement in daily activities such as when lifting objects or bending over.

7. **Shorten the lever.**

   When hip hinging, flexing, or extending your spine, keep your arms out to your sides or alongside your body to reduce the load placed on the muscles of your lower back. Bend your elbows instead of using straight arms. Any position can be used as long as your arms are not lifted next to the ears with elbows fully extended. This position, for many, creates more stress in the shoulder and neck area. For example, when moving from standing forward fold (see part II) back to mountain pose (see part II), sweep your arms around and up instead of reaching directly forward. Or, in locust pose (see part II), keep your arms back alongside your body instead of in front of you.

- **Mats or blankets.** Place a mat or blanket under your head, knees, or lower back for support in positions in which you lie on your back. You can also sit on a rolled-up mat or folded blanket to lift your hips in seated forward folds to maintain a straight spine.
- **Walls.** Use a wall for support during standing balances and simple inversions.
- **Kneepads.** If you have sensitive knees, place a folded towel under your kneecaps, or cut an old yoga mat into strips to place over your mat for extra padding during kneeling poses.

## Other Items

Yoga is a personal experience. Create an environment for your practice that invites you back. You can do so in many ways. Some suggestions are offered here, but have fun experimenting with what motivates or inspires you to make your workout feel as if you're coming home.

### Music

Although some people opt not to play music so that they can focus only on the sound of their breathing, a good CD or playlist that matches the tone of your practice is often helpful for inspiration and motivation. Music is also a powerful tool in helping you relax and shifting you into slower brain wave (healing and calming) states faster.

YogaFit provides many options for music so that you can find a style that suits you and your workout, from ambient music without lyrics (to energize without distracting) to a variety of styles and mixes with vocals (to lighten or enhance the tone while motivating). Many CDs and playlists in more active or Zen-like styles are formatted to match the three mountains of a YogaFit workout (see chapter 4). They begin with slower music, progress to more upbeat music in the middle, and then wind down in tempo for deep stretches and final relaxation. Using these CDs, you need not switch out your music in the middle of your practice. YogaFit has a large selection of music on CDs and digital downloads to satisfy a wide variety of tastes. You can check out the current selection at www.yogafit.com.

### Aromatherapy

Natural essential oils in a diffuser create a pleasing setting and a scent awareness during your YogaFit session. If you haven't used essential oils and want to try, stick to the basics to help you get started. Use only certified therapeutic grade oils so that you can be sure they contain no fillers or impurities in the oil. You can find these oils and more information about the use and benefits of essential oils online at www.mydoterra.com/yogafit/index.html. Please check with your doctor about your use of essential oils in the case of allergic response or sensitivity to certain plants.

Here are just a few examples of commonly used oils:

- *Lavender* is one of the most commonly used oils and has many therapeutic uses. Inhaling lavender oil has a soothing and relaxing effect on the mind. Studies show that it quickly activates the parasympathetic nervous system (also known as the rest-and-digest system)—perfect for winding down after a hard day.

- *Eucalyptus* is widely known for its calming effect and has been shown to reduce feelings of anxiety. Eucalyptus oil can increase mental clarity while helping the muscles relax, making it a great companion on the mat. Add several drops to a spray bottle with water, and you have a wonderful natural mat cleaner.

- *Wild orange* is an invigorating, uplifting oil that creates a warm, happy feeling when inhaled. Wild orange is one the most powerful oils, supporting the immune system in eliminating toxins from the body and stimulating the lymphatic system. Wild orange is great for a morning practice, leaving you feeling energized yet peaceful. What a great way to start you day!

- *Ylang ylang* has a beautiful floral scent and is known to relax your mind, lift your spirits, and perhaps lower blood pressure caused by stress. Use this oil when practicing restorative yoga.

- *Sandalwood* has been used for over 4,000 years in Hindu ceremonies and is still used today for medicinal purposes, to calm nerves, and to decrease anxiety.

- *Patchouli,* a beautiful scent with hints of orange and amber, reduces anxiety and relaxes your mind.

### Candles

Candles give an ambient glow and can provide a focal point that is beneficial for standing balance poses. Use soy candles that burn without toxic fumes (see appendix B).

# Special Considerations for YogaFit

Special conditions such as pregnancy, injury, or other medical conditions may require you to modify your YogaFit sessions. Note that inverted poses and backbends are for advanced students after a vigorous warm-up only.

## Injuries or Medical Conditions

Here is a list of common injuries and medical conditions for which you will likely need to modify your YogaFit workout:

- *Sciatica.* Bend your knees in forward folds. Avoid intense hamstring stretches.

- *Hypertension (high blood pressure).* Avoid holding your breath; avoid inverted postures.

- *Glaucoma or other eye problems.* Avoid holding your breath; avoid inverted postures.

- *Sinus infections, ear infections, congestion.* Avoid holding your breath; avoid inverted postures.

- *Back or neck injuries.* Avoid inverted postures.
- *Knee problems.* Pay special attention to alignment of the knees in poses that stretch the quads and standing postures keeping hips, knees and toes in alignment; do the upside-down pigeon with extra care. Use kneepads or place extra padding under the knees for floor work.
- *Wrist injuries or painful conditions such as carpal tunnel.* Make "fists" for wrists (palms facing each other) in any pose in which shoulders are stacked directly above the wrists, such as incline plank, cat and cow, spinal balance, or tabletop. Using fists for wrists is not an option in downward-facing dog, so an alternative pose such as dolphin pose or child's pose is a good choice.
- *Shoulder injuries.* Avoid raising your arms for extended periods, such as in warrior II or chair. Also avoid poses that place a heavy load on your shoulders, such as the crocodile and plank poses, or drop your knees when performing these poses. Also keep hands directly under pectorals in crocodile or plank poses to support your shoulders.

## Pregnancy

Although yoga is wonderful for prenatal conditioning, pregnant women should consult their doctors before beginning a YogaFit practice, as they would for any exercise program. Here are some key points for pregnant women to keep in mind:

- Women who are used to performing regular exercise will experience a decline in performance during pregnancy. This decline is natural and unavoidable, and you should not try to compensate for it. In fact, because you have less oxygen available for aerobic exercise, you need to limit the intensity of your session and lower your target heart rate.
- Avoid overstretching. Hormonal changes cause ligaments to loosen, and going too deeply into a posture can result in injury. Pay special attention to core stability to protect the joints and connective tissue when practicing for two. Also avoid lower spinal twists, low lunges, upward facing dog, and supine-lying poses. Use caution with poses such as warrior I (it can create pressure in the SI joints and low back), forward folds (seated or standing; legs should be spaced apart to allow room for your growing abdomen), child's pose (space knees apart to allow room for your growing abdomen), and backbends like camel to avoid putting too much stretch on the abdomen.
- Avoid prolonged inverted postures, and refrain from holding your breath; they can limit the flow of blood to the fetus. In addition, pregnancy might affect circulation, so be sure to keep warm (but overheating is also dangerous for the fetus, so dress in layers). After the first trimester, avoid prolonged periods of standing or lying flat on your back.
- Body changes remain for 4 to 6 weeks after pregnancy. New mothers should be careful not to overextend themselves. Take time to gradually work back into your regular fitness routine.

YogaFit poses can be modified to accommodate the physical changes in pregnant women's bodies. For example, in the third trimester a wall or chair can be used to aid balance. For more information on safely continuing your YogaFit practice during pregnancy and beyond, look for YogaFit's manual and DVDs for prenatal and postpartum, which can be purchased at www.yogafit.com.

## Seniors

It is never too late to begin a YogaFit practice. YogaFit is one of the best exercise formats for older adults, but anyone 65 and older should consult a doctor before beginning a YogaFit practice. Here are key points for seniors to keep in mind:

- YogaFit for seniors is based on simple, repetitive movements. Older yoga students can derive enormous benefits from such movements when they are combined with breathing techniques. In fact, the single most important point of focus in a YogaFit class for seniors is deep breathing.

- If you're over 65, begin each session with an extended warm-up (as is done in YogaFit classes for seniors), and take more time to focus on your breathing, shoulder-opening poses (such as chest expansion), and balance. Some poses can be done sitting in a chair, or while standing and using a chair or wall for support. At the end of your session, allow at least 10 minutes for final relaxation. You may want to consider purchasing YogaFit's *YogaFit Seniors DVD Vol. 2*.

- The older yoga student should initially avoid certain poses, including extended periods of inversion (especially seniors with high blood pressure, glaucoma, or cataracts), extended periods of floor postures or forward flexion, and complex postures that require a lot of strength. Older students should pay special attention to spinal alignment to ensure safe transitions into and out of the poses.

Again, check with your doctor about which poses are appropriate for you and when. For more information on YogaFit for seniors, look for YogaFit's manual and DVDs for seniors at www.yogafit.com.

## Time to Begin

As necessary, return to this chapter for review. The more you know about YogaFit, and the more consistently you practice, the greater the benefits you'll receive. Remember to start where you are and be patient with your progress. Even 5 minutes of deep breathing today is better than waiting one more day to start. Most important, remember to have fun!

# CHAPTER 3

# YogaFit Breathing

Breath is life. You breathe in oxygen, and your amazing body delivers this life-sustaining nourishment to the cells. Most people don't think about breathing because it is automatic. However, how you breathe can have a major impact on your health. YogaFit instructors often give these instructions: *We don't move without breathing, and we don't breathe without moving.* In yoga, you bring attention to your breath, specifically, deepening and the slowing the breath. Ancient yogic text tells that swimming is the closest thing to yogic breathing—slow, strong, steady, long breaths. Yogis have known the amazing benefits of breathing practices for thousands of years, but scientists in the Western world have only recently established a clear connection between deep, controlled breathing and improved health. A study reported in the *International Journal of Yoga Therapy* in 2011 showed that just 5 minutes of slow, deep breathing (6 breaths per minute) reduced heart rate and blood pressure in hypertensive patients (Bhavanani et al. 2011). One of the greatest health benefits of conscious breathing is stress reduction. It is well known that stress is linked to a number of health conditions, including high blood pressure, heart disease, and depression. Just learning how to breathe deeply and with more attention both on and off the mat can reduce (and even eliminate) many of the symptoms triggered by stress.

In traditional yoga, the breath is known to drive and direct *prana,* or the universal life-force energy within everyone. Thus, your pranic body is your vital body, also known as pranamaya kosha (your energy body, discussed in chapter 1). Everything is energy in one form or another. You breathe in the universal energy (prana), and through the practice of pranayama you learn to control your individual energy (called *vasti prana*) and how it flows through the body. Classic yogic breathing techniques are known as *pranayama,* or practices created to control the breath and harness the prana within and surrounding your body in order to create a state of inner peace. Your pranic energy moves throughout your body in various directions. If you are stiff and tight or holding tension anywhere, then that energy is unable to flow freely. One way to describe prana and its movement is to say it corresponds to the left and right side of your body. Your right side is associated with increased

**More than ever, people need to pay attention to the way they are breathing. The increased oxygen you breathe in from conscious, deep breathing gives you more physical energy and improves concentration and mental clarity, which is one of the first things people lose when under stress. To increase your oxygen levels, focus on breathing deeply all the way to your navel rather than only to your upper chest.**

energy, heat, and alertness. Your left side is associated with internal awareness, cooling, and calm. Optimum health is about balancing these energies. If your pranic energy is blocked or out of balance, then the result will be disease in some form. More than breath control exercises, then, pranayama is about controlling the life force. It is said in the ancient yogic texts that the practice of physical postures helps unblock obstructions in the body, and the practice of pranayama regulates the flow of prana, which is linked to the regulation of the mind and the actions. Ancient yogis who understood the essence of prana studied pranayama and devised methods and practices to master it—many of which YogaFit teaches and are provided in this chapter.

YogaFit breathing and pranayama practices offer these benefits as well:

- Increased strength and control of the diaphragm (primary breathing muscle) and other core muscles
- Increased heat and energy
- Heightened awareness, concentration, and control
- Increased control of prana for physical and mental balance
- Decreased anxiety
- Deep relaxation for the body and mind

People take between 10 and 16 breaths per minute during normal daily activities and about 6 to 8 breaths per minute while at rest. It's common during everyday life to use only the upper third of your lungs. This kind of shallow breathing is generally caused by tension or stress and sometimes postural problems. People with excessive kyphosis (rounded upper back) are known to have shorter life spans than people without it. It's nearly impossible to take a deep breath while in a slumping posture. Because the blood vessels are more plentiful in the lower lobes of the lungs, you need to use your entire lung capacity in order to get enough oxygen into the body, and to release the toxins eliminated as you exhale. The modern lifestyle of sitting, computer work, driving, and texting is sometimes referred to as a ***forward-flexion lifestyle,*** meaning the front of the body is closed off, reducing the ability to breathe deeply.

Once you begin to practice deep breathing regularly, you'll experience for yourself the profound impact your breath has on your mental and physical energy and on your well-being.

In YogaFit, when moving from one pose to the next, you match the flow of the poses to the pace of your deepest breath (vinyasa). Although you often hold certain poses and breathe through them, at no point do you move without breathing. Remember to find your own perfect pace, trusting that with practice your breath and movement will synchronize effortlessly, making both easier.

# YogaFit Breath

The breathing techniques described in this chapter are essential to the YogaFit lifestyle. You'll use them in every YogaFit session for the most powerful and effective mental and physical experience.

## Nose Breathing

Traditional yoga breathing practices are done exclusively through the nose. YogaFit teaches nose breathing because breaths taken in through your nose warm, humidify, and filter the air coming into your body. These breaths keep your body warmer while you work out, which is necessary for your muscles and connective tissue to stretch safely and effectively. Breathing through your nose also demands greater concentration, which helps you stay focused and connected with your body during even the most challenging phases of your practice. Finally, nose breathing is more efficient for your heart and lungs, which is why many professional athletes practice this technique.

### Nose Breathing Exercise

Each of the following breathing practices relies on nose breathing. Practice by sitting tall, either while cross-legged on the floor or in a chair, or by lying on your back. Close your lips, and breathe deeply through your nose. What do you notice about the quality of your breath? How does nose breathing make you feel?

## Ujjayi Breath

Like nose breathing, you'll use a yoga technique called *ujjayi* breath (meaning "victorious breath") in every YogaFit session. The only time you won't use ujjayi breath is during final relaxation. This technique is also used in conjunction with other pranayama techniques, as will be described. The purpose of ujjayi is to make your breath audible, yet not too loud—just loud enough for you alone to hear. This breath allows you to monitor both the quality and quantity of your breath as you work out. If you can hear your breath, you'll recognize when it's becoming rapid and shallow or whether it's staying steady and deep. Ujjayi also gives you a focal point when your mind begins to wander. Ujjayi and other resonant breathing techniques have a calming effect on the nervous system.

Ujjayi breathing requires you to partially close your glottis (the part in your throat that closes when you swallow but is open when you breathe). Breathing this way creates a whispery sound, which is why the technique is also termed *whisper breath*. Ujjayi breathing can be compared to the sound Darth Vader makes in Star Wars, though not quite as amplified. If there is too much effort (force) used to create the sound, then you will feel tension develop. The goal is to find the softness and ease, both of which come with practice.

## Ujjayi Breath Exercise

Practice by sitting tall, either cross-legged on the floor or in a chair, or by lying on your back. Close your lips, and breathe deeply through your nose. Begin ujjayi breathing, focusing on matching the quality and quantity of every inhalation to every exhalation. Once you have mastered this technique at rest, try it when under stress or exertion, such as when driving in traffic or riding your bicycle.

## Three-Part Breath

The three-part breath, also known as the complete breath, is the simplest and most rewarding of all yogic breathing exercises. It is both purifying and energizing, and, if done slowly and evenly, it can produce a sense of serenity and balance. As mentioned, in daily life people often breathe with only the top portion of the lungs, neglecting to get the oxygen needed in order to function at their full potential. Thus, breathing in and out at full capacity even just a few times can markedly increase blood oxygen levels and decrease carbon dioxide. Three-part breaths are great for heightening your awareness of your breathing from moment to moment and helping you recognize—and use—the potential depth of your lungs.

In a three-part breath you use your diaphragm to fill your lungs completely from bottom to top. To practice this technique, first focus on expanding your belly, then your ribs, and then your chest, before exhaling completely. It can be helpful when you first start to practice to place the hands on the belly, then the ribs and then the chest, and have the breath follow the hands. Three-part breaths can be used at any time in a YogaFit session, including at the beginning and end of your session with relaxation breath (discussed next). Three-part breathing is usually coupled with ujjayi breathing for greater awareness and control.

## Three-Part Breath Exercise

Sit tall and inhale, bringing your breath deep into your abdomen, then rib cage, and finally into your chest and throat. Exhale slowly and completely, letting everything go. Repeat several times.

## Relaxation Breath

Relaxation breath is a slow-paced technique used to induce a state of deep relaxation and centeredness. Sometimes called belly breath, it's the simplest and easiest method of breathing. Everyone should practice it under the pressure and rush of daily life, because it helps reverse the physiological symptoms of stress, including lowering the heart rate and decreasing blood pressure. Although a relaxation breath is not as deep as a three-part breath, this technique also focuses on matching the length and depth of the inhalation to that of the exhalation. Use relaxation breath during the first pose of your warm-up and in your final relaxation pose in order to achieve a serene, restorative state.

### Relaxation Breath Exercise

Lying comfortably on your back, relax completely. Place your right hand on your chest and your left hand on the upper part of your abdomen. Breathe so that only your left hand rises during the inhalation and falls during the exhalation. Your right hand remains virtually motionless. Give an equal amount of time to the inhalation and the exhalation. Breathing this way should never be a struggle. Do only what you're able to do calmly and comfortably.

## Sinking Breath

People know that trying to force flexibility causes the muscles to resist and shorten. Sinking breath is a technique that uses longer exhalations to move you gently into a deeper stretch. By extending your exhalation in poses that move toward the center of the earth (e.g., standing forward fold; downward-facing dog; or pyramid), your muscles relax, release, and lengthen.

### Sinking Breath Exercise

Assume a relaxed pose such as child's pose or forward fold. Inhaling, feel your body lift slightly. As you exhale slowly and completely, allow your body to sink more deeply into the pose. Repeat sinking breaths for the duration of your pose (see chapter 4).

## Expanding Breath

Expanding breath focuses on your inhalations. It is used in poses that open your chest to the sky (e.g., standing backbend, camel, bridge, or triangle). On every inhalation you breathe in deeply, lifting and expanding your chest; you then maintain that expansiveness as you exhale. An open chest allows you to breathe more deeply. The effort required to hold your chest open builds strength and support in and around your spine.

## Expanding Breath Exercise

Assume a relaxed pose, such as chest expansion or kneeling camel pose, and inhale, filling your lungs deeply with air. As your chest expands, be aware of how your whole body lifts and opens as you take this breath. Keep that open feeling even while you exhale. Repeat this expanding breath for the duration of your pose (see chapter 4).

# Locks

*Bandha* is a Sanskrit term that means "lock." A lock binds the physical body to the vital (energetic) body. The practice of pranayama helps to harness prana and control its flow. You can enhance this prana with a bandha, a defined area within your anatomy activated through muscular contraction.

Many locks are practiced in traditional yoga, but this program focuses on two primary locks that are used in hatha yoga: root lock (called *mula bandha*) and belly lock (called *uddiyana bandha*). As you try some exercises to develop awareness, you might discover that you already know how to apply a bandha.

## Root Lock

The root lock is about grounding. It involves a gentle, firm contraction of the pelvic floor muscles, activating your inner thighs and core to stabilize your pose. Root lock can also involve centering your thoughts on gaining ground and maintaining your status or standing in life. Finally, as it relates to prana, root lock is often combined with pranayama techniques.

## Root Lock Exercise

Root lock is the contraction of three small muscles within the perineum. Picture the base of your pelvis as a diamond, with a line drawn horizontally across the middle to create two triangles. The upper triangle is the perineum. The lower triangle is the anal sphincter muscle, which should remain relaxed. One way to explain root lock is comparing it to how it feels to stop your flow of urination. This is the sensation you feel when you contract your perineum.

## Belly Lock

Belly lock is about creating and storing energy. It can increase your energy level, cleanse and stimulate your digestive system, and increase your lung capacity by stretching your diaphragm for deeper, more efficient breathing.

Belly lock is always combined with root lock. It involves the abdominals, diaphragm, and intercostal muscles (muscles between the ribs). Belly lock can be performed as a core-stabilizing exercise or as a breath-holding technique.

Either way, make sure you're comfortable with sustained breath retention after exhaling before performing the belly lock while holding your breath.

## Belly Lock Exercise

Begin by inhaling to fill your lungs. While exhaling, draw your abdominal muscles inward and upward to empty your lungs completely. At the end of your exhalation, tuck your chin into your chest as if you were holding a small tennis ball under your chin. If practicing breath retention, hold your breath out to create a vacuum-like energy that draws your organs up, holding them against your diaphragm. To avoid gasping, release your abdomen and chin before inhaling. Practice belly lock as you perform these pranayama techniques:

- Lying-down three-part breath
- Seated three-part breath

Note your experience in each technique. Remember that belly lock builds on root lock, so contract your perineum before and during each of the exercises.

In chapter 1, you learned the YogaFit essence and the importance of letting go when learning any aspect of yoga. These ideas apply to the poses as well as the breath. While breathing practices are about controlling prana, they are only effective when approached without expectation, competition, and judgment. Stay in the present, embrace the process of taking in and letting out each breath, and delight in what conscious breathing can effect in your life.

# CHAPTER 4

# Three Mountains of YogaFit

 YogaFit applies modern exercise science to the ancient mind–body practice of yoga. Although yoga can have a profound impact on the physical, emotional, and spiritual health of students, improper sequencing and pacing creates opportunities for physical discomfort and injury. For this reason, YogaFit classes follow a format called the three mountains. This format is consistent with current group exercise standards and guidelines for the safest, most effective, and consistent progression possible. YogaFit has followed this format since 1995, training over 500,000 people worldwide in the powerful YogaFit style.

YogaFit works from the gross to the subtle, warming up the largest muscle groups and joints first and working toward smaller groups. By the time you get to complex postures, your body is warm and ready to be there.

Every workout begins by preparing your body in two ways. First, you create heat by working the large muscle groups through a gentle range of motion to lubricate the joints, an important factor that helps reduce the chances of injury. This preparation allows the muscles and connective tissue to later stretch safely, without injury. (See chapter 9 for details on safe stretching and flexibility.) As the body warms up you can begin to move in an increasing range of motion, which prepares the body for more intense strength work and stretching while increasing muscular endurance. In mountain I of a YogaFit class, you follow these guidelines by flowing (moving) in and out of the poses continuously to build heat while introducing your muscles and joints gently to the positions you will hold in mountain II. Mountain I also provides an opportunity to check in with the body and notice whether any parts need a little more attention and care in this practice. Each time you step on your mat, your practice is going to be unique depending on both our state of mind and your degree of physical activity the day before.

**"Any yoga is good yoga as long as it is safe yoga."**

Range of motion involves more than muscles. Genetic bone structure and the health of your joints also determine how flexible you are or can become. To avoid injury and get the most out of your yoga practice, relax and move only as far as you are comfortable, and match your breath with your movement. Be open to exploring different variations of the poses in each practice so that you can find the best position for that day.

After you warm up (mountain I), the focus turns to strength, endurance, flexibility, and balance. According to fitness guidelines, people achieve strength and endurance by progressively overloading the muscle with increasing workload and range of motion and moving a muscle several times through a specific range of motion. In mountain II, you do both. Most of the poses are held in isometric contraction to build strength, yet flows are often inserted in order to increase endurance. (See the section titled Flow Series later in this chapter). Further, the variety of poses YogaFit offers ensures that every major muscle is targeted in every class (and most minor muscles, too), maximizing your strength while maintaining balance.

Every workout should end with a cool-down. YogaFit's mountain III brings you down to your mat for poses that focus on deep stretches held for longer periods of time to increase flexibility, lower the heart rate, and deliver a profound sense of relaxation. As you work into mountain III, you are decreasing the intensity of the workout and moving toward the final phase of any healthy fitness regimen, rest and recovery.

YogaFit's three-mountain format consists of these three phases:

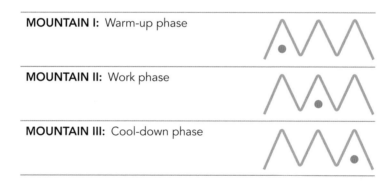

**MOUNTAIN I:** Warm-up phase

**MOUNTAIN II:** Work phase

**MOUNTAIN III:** Cool-down phase

YogaFit also includes these two valley phases, which are extensions of mountain I and mountain II:

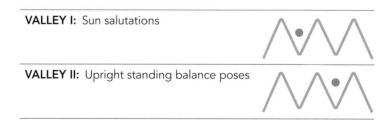

**VALLEY I:** Sun salutations

**VALLEY II:** Upright standing balance poses

**Flow Series**

The flow series, also called the half series, is a dynamic flow of four poses that comprises the "bottom" half of the sun salutation, YogaFit's valley I series. You use this flow to help warm up the body in mountain I and valley I, and you use it to retain heat in mountain II.

In mountain I, you begin with the modified version of this series: This version warms up the larger muscle groups in the upper body by moving the joints and spine through their natural ranges of motion. It also prepares you for the next stage of the workout, valley I (sun salutations), in which poses are added to the series and the more challenging option of coming off the knees is introduced.

In mountain II the body is warm and prepared for the work phase of the practice. Inserting the flow series between the standing poses and the standing pose sequences has several benefits:

- It keeps your body warm.
- It builds upper-body and core strength.
- It increases endurance.
- It strengthens the cardiovascular system.
- It promotes musculoskeletal balance.

You can do the flow series on or off the knees, depending on your strength and ability. Both options target the same muscles. If you are a beginner, you can start on the knees until you have the strength to practice the series off your knees without struggling or dropping your hips and belly, such as might occur in a plank or crocodile pose. When the flow series is first introduced in mountain I, for safety you omit cobra (a backbend) until your muscles have warmed up more. Repeat the series as often as you like in mountain I as a warm-up or in mountain II between standing pose sequences. (Chapter 10 presents several workouts that include the flow series.) Again, the number of repetitions is up to you, as long as you're listening to your body. Doing this half series flow in the warm-up helps to build a good foundation with correct alignment in the shoulders and a strong core.

Here are the sequences for the modified flow series (kneeling) and the flow series (standing):

**Modified Flow Series (Kneeling)**

Child's pose

Kneeling plank

Kneeling crocodile

Cobra (omit in mountain I)

Child's pose

**Flow Series (Standing)**

Downward-facing dog

Plank

Crocodile

Upward-facing dog

Downward-facing dog

# Mountain I: Warm-Up Phase

Before you begin mountain I, the warm-up phase for YogaFit, start with 3 to 5 minutes of deep breathing (see chapter 3) to help you get centered in your body. This deep breathing oxygenates the blood, warms the body, and creates focus for your session.

After deep breathing, begin moving through one of two warm-ups in chapter 10. In mountain I, you always flow through the poses with your breath. In other words, you inhale into one pose and exhale into the next. As a general rule, inhaling is paired with an opening move (e.g., inhaling while sweeping the arms up to the sky), and exhaling is paired with a closing move (e.g., exhaling into forward fold). Often you'll repeat a pose several times, using each phase of your breath to take you in and out of the posture. Movements are done through the large muscle groups (quadriceps, hamstrings, gluteal muscles, and back muscles), using the large joints of the body (knees, shoulders, hips, elbows, and spine). These movements help to warm your body, increase heart rate, and promote muscular elasticity. If you're sweating during this phase, it's a good thing.

# Valley I: Sun Salutations

In yoga, a salutation is a series of poses with a specific focus or purpose. In YogaFit, the sun salutations complete your warm-up phase by working all major muscles and joints through a greater range of motion. Sun salutations flow one breath per movement so that heat continues to build as you prepare for mountain II.

Sun salutations are sequential and always flow in the same order. In valley I, the sequence is repeated on the right and left sides of the body at least twice. Remember that you can modify sun salutations by using the kneeling version (modified flow series). Here is the sequence of a sun salutation (with breath cues in parentheses):

- Mountain (*inhale*)
- Standing forward fold (*exhale*)
- Crescent lunge or kneeling lunge (*inhale*)
- Downward-facing dog or child's pose (*exhale*)
- Plank or kneeling plank (*inhale*)
- Crocodile or kneeling crocodile (*exhale*)
- Upward-facing dog or cobra (*inhale*)
- Downward-facing dog or child's pose (*exhale*)
- Crescent lunge or kneeling lunge (*inhale*)
- Standing forward fold (*exhale*)
- Mountain (*inhale*)
- Chair (*exhale*)

# Mountain II: Work Phase

Mountain II poses are listed in the workouts in chapter 10. Mountain II is the work phase of your YogaFit session. In this phase you can use the heat built in mountain I and valley I to work into standing poses that build strength, endurance, and flexibility for the upper and lower body. Poses in mountain II use lunging positions to build strength and flexibility in the lower body, and arm and torso positions for strength and flexibility in the upper body. Because your muscles are warm, they are now responsive to this type of movement.

Holding poses for three to five breaths on each side in mountain II helps strengthen the muscles through isometric contraction, or through engaging a muscle or muscle group while holding it in one position. As the postures become more challenging, use three-part breath or ujjayi breath (see chapter 3) to aid concentration and provide energy. Always take a break when you need one.

# Valley II: Upright Standing Balance Poses

Valley II poses are listed in chapter 6. In valley II, standing balance poses are practiced with the head above the heart. Performing these poses at this point has two primary benefits: first, to improve overall balance and muscular coordination and second, to allow your blood pressure to equalize in the upper and lower halves of your body. Equalizing your blood pressure before coming down to the floor will prevent a drop in blood pressure that could lead to dizziness or even fainting.

Poses in valley II are held for 5 to 10 breaths on each side. Practice as many as you like in any order that you choose.

# Mountain III: Cool-Down Phase

Mountain III poses are listed in chapters 7, 8, and 9. Mountain III is the cool-down phase of your YogaFit session. In this phase, you use the heat created in mountain II to move deeper into prone (on your belly), seated, and supine (on your back) poses to build strength and flexibility through deep stretching. Seated and prone poses are usually reserved for mountain III for the sake of flow. Once you come down to the floor, you can relax in the idea that you don't have to get back up until you have completed the practice. While some mountain III poses build strength, most offer opportunities for deep stretching and release.

To build flexibility, hold mountain III poses for 5 to 10 breaths on each side. Holding poses for 30 to 45 seconds or more allows muscles to retain length and promotes release of muscle tension.

Note that every YogaFit session ends with 6 to 10 minutes in the final relaxation pose, during which you begin to physically and mentally integrate the benefits of your workout. This final phase provides an important transition from your practice back into your daily routine. See chapter 9 for more information on the final relaxation pose and its benefits.

Final relaxation is characterized by deep relaxation with an easy breathing pattern that promotes a meditative and potentially healing state. Because stress and stress-related conditions and illnesses are so prevalent, and because people often don't take enough time to rest, this part of your session is critical for restoration and healing. Some people actually find spending time quietly in relaxation more challenging than the poses themselves. If this is true for you, you might benefit more from this phase of the session than from any other. Give yourself the time and space to relax and enjoy the benefits of your practice. Yoga was designed to ready the body for meditation, so at least relax and enjoy the fruits of your labors. Final relaxation—*ahhhhhh*.

PART **II**

# Purposeful Poses

# CHAPTER 5

# Core Strength and Stability

The term *core* is a buzzword in the fitness industry, and for good reason. A strong midsection, including the abdominal, gluteal, and lower-back muscles, is helpful in many areas, including deep breathing and improved efficiency, balance, and athletic performance. Conditioning your core also helps prevent back pain and injury.

Working your core does far more than just build strong muscles. When your core is strong, you feel strong. A powerful midsection enhances the qualities of the third chakra (solar plexus), strengthening willpower, personal power, determination, and discipline (see appendix A).

Nearly all the YogaFit poses increase core strength and stability. Whether you're standing, balancing, twisting, or inverting, you use your core to keep you steady. This chapter focuses on poses that target your midsection.

As noted in chapter 2, creating core stability is one of YogaFit's seven principles of alignment (SPA). In chapter 3, you learned about two locks—root lock and belly lock. For this discussion two secondary locks, foot lock (called *pada bandha* in Sanskrit) and hand lock (called *hasta bandha* in Sanskrit) are added, because they relate to your ability to ground your poses (see figures 5.1 *a* and *b*). In standing poses, core activation actually begins in your feet with the lifting of the arches as you establish your base. This action is the foot lock. The muscles that lift the arches of the feet are connected through fascia (connective tissue) to the muscles of the lower leg, the adductors (inner thigh), the pelvic floor (activating mula bandha), the transverse abdominal muscles (activating uddiyana bandha), the diaphragm, the trapezius muscles (upper-back muscles), and all the way up to the neck flexors. When you activate pada bandha (foot lock), the resulting contraction of muscles up the kinetic chain (legs, pelvic floor, deep abdominal muscles, and spinal muscles are all connected and movement in one area affects the rest of the chain) helps to keep your joints soft (unlocked), and because it connects to

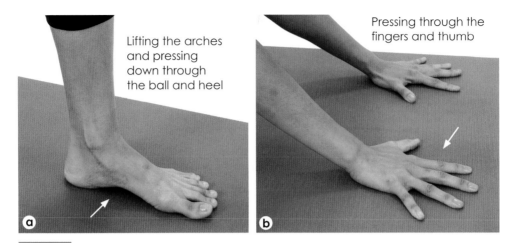

**Figure 5.1**    *(a)* Foot lock and *(b)* hand lock.

mula bandha (root lock) and uddiyana bandha (belly lock), it helps keep the spine in alignment. The dynamic tension created by the isometric contraction of the muscles helps in achieving and maintaining alignment along the entire kinetic chain because of the layers of fascia surrounding the muscles. Experts no longer think about movement as separate muscles that are contracting in isolation. In the last 10 years research has shown that fascia throughout the body serves to link the entire body together. This concept is important when you apply it to moving because if you have tightness in one area of the body, other areas and movement will be affected. The beauty of a YogaFit practice is that you are moving in so many planes with the addition of deep breathing that you are able to make changes in the body rather quickly.

> A core muscle people often neglect to target in workouts is the diaphragm, the dome-shaped muscle that separates your chest cavity and lungs from your abdominal area, where most vital organs are located. The diaphragm is your primary breathing muscle. Because your circulatory, respiratory, and nervous systems are all affected by your ability to take a deep breath, you need to regularly exercise your diaphragm. YogaFit's three-part breath, along with other breathing exercises described in chapter 3, targets the diaphragm.

# Connecting Breath With Core and Bandhas: Bandha Breathing

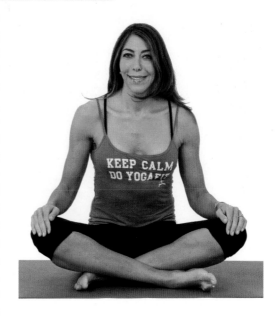

Practicing this breathing technique will help you avoid becoming too rigid in the activation of the bandhas. In an easy seated pose with the spine in neutral (elevate the hips if the back is rounded), begin deep diaphragmatic breathing. Notice the sensation of the inhalation and the exhalation. After about five breaths, on the exhalation activate mula bandha and uddiyana bandha (draw the pelvic floor muscles up toward the heart and hug the energy toward the center of your body). Then on the inhalation release both bandhas. After you get comfortable with the activation and the release, begin to play around with different intensities of contraction and release so that you find the place where as you exhale, you contract about 80 percent; and on the inhalation, you release to about 20 percent contraction. Look for an easy flow that you will be able to find again in any pose. This ebb and flow of bandha contraction and energy will help you to be able to find mobility and stability within your practice. You can also practice this connection in mountain pose or seated in a chair.

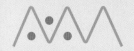

# Plank and Kneeling Plank

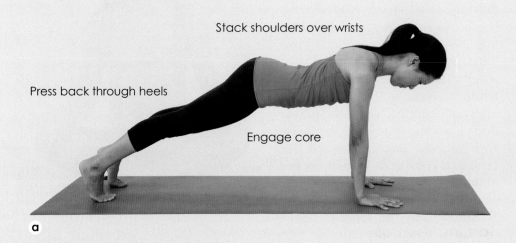

Stack shoulders over wrists

Press back through heels

Engage core

a

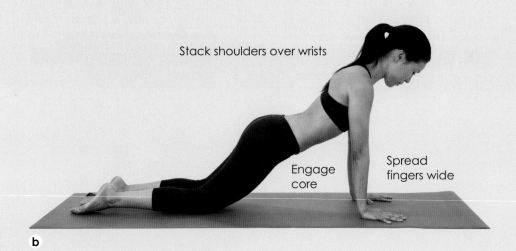

Stack shoulders over wrists

Engage core

Spread fingers wide

b

On or off the knees, plank pose works many major muscles of the upper body and core. Use this pose in mountains I and II and in sun salutations (valley I).

## Getting Into the Pose

**Plank (figure *a*):** From downward-facing dog, shift forward until your shoulders are directly above your wrists. Press your heels back toward the wall behind you. Reach forward through the crown of your head. Keep your back straight and abdominal muscles firm.

**Kneeling plank (figure *b*):** From child's pose, shift forward until your shoulders are directly above your wrists. Keep your back straight and abdominal muscles firm.

## Holding the Pose

In mountain II, you can pause and hold the plank or kneeling plank pose for three to five breaths. Keep your body aligned, hips slightly elevated. In mountain I or valley I, move through plank or kneeling plank as part of the flow series or sun salutations. To deepen the sensation, try lifting the arches of the feet (pada bandha) while keeping the center of the chest reaching forward. Notice a little more activity in the deep core.

## Modification

If you're a beginner or if your midsection sags in plank pose, practice kneeling plank.

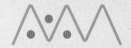

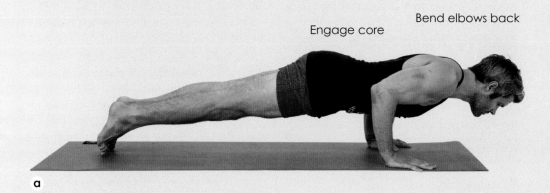

Engage core

Bend elbows back

**a**

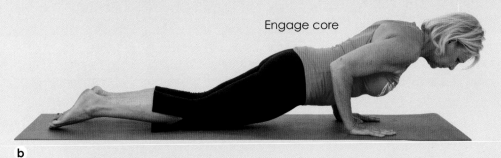

Bend elbows back

Engage core

**b**

**STRENGTHENS:**
abdominal muscles • lower back •
chest • shoulders • triceps

Use crocodile pose after plank and kneeling plank poses to work the upper body and core in mountains I and II, as well as in sun salutations (valley I). Lower into crocodile pose as you exhale, moving directly into cobra or upward-facing dog (see Pose Index for location of poses) on the next inhalation.

## Getting Into the Pose

**Crocodile (figure *a*):** From plank pose, push forward with your toes, pressing through the fingers. Lower your chest, keeping your abdominal muscles strong and hips stationary. To keep your shoulders safe, avoid lowering your shoulders below your elbows.

**Kneeling crocodile (figure *b*):** From kneeling plank, shift forward, bringing your shoulders over your fingertips. Press your fingers firmly into the mat to stabilize while lowering your torso, keeping your abdominal muscles strong supporting the spine.

## Modification

If you're a beginner or if your midsection sags in crocodile pose, practice kneeling crocodile pose.

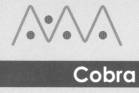

# Cobra

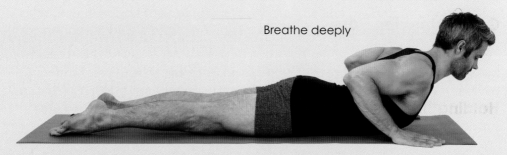

Focus on lengthening

Breathe deeply

Of all the backbending postures in yoga, the ones done on the belly are the most popular. Practice cobra pose for a strong, supple back and open chest. Cobra pose follows kneeling crocodile in mountains I and II, as well as in valley I as part of sun salutations. Because you're already down on the floor, you can also use cobra in mountain III. Before you begin, review the introduction to chapter 7 for information on safe and effective backbending.

## Getting Into the Pose

From your belly, rest your hands lightly on the floor next to your chest. Use your back to lift your chest up and forward. Draw your shoulders back and down.

## Holding the Pose

Keep the back of your neck long and your lower body strong. Without pushing with your hands, lengthen your torso as you lift. In mountain I (after warming up) or valley I, move through cobra pose as part of the modified flow series or sun salutations. In mountain II hold for 3 to 5 breaths; in mountain III hold for 5 to 10 breaths. The challenge of lifting away from the floor against the pull of gravity is offset by the ease of exiting the backbend. Release slowly, and push back to child's pose.

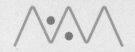

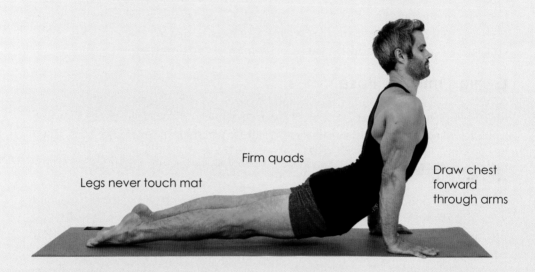

Firm quads

Legs never touch mat

Draw chest forward through arms

Upward-facing dog pose is part of the flow series, but it is also a backbend. Use this pose in mountain II and in valley I to stretch the front of your body and strengthen the muscles of your lower body and back. Before you begin, check chapter 7 for information on safe and effective backbending.

## Getting Into the Pose

From crocodile pose, place the tops of your feet on the floor and straighten your arms. Pull your chest up and forward, keeping your lower back long and your abdominal muscles strong.

## Holding the Pose

In mountain II, pause and hold upward-facing dog for three to five breaths. Continue to draw your body forward, engaging the muscles in your lower legs and buttocks. Keep your elbows unlocked and your shoulders away from your ears. For a deepening sensation, press through the length of the fingers and the thumb as if your hands were suction cups. This action is called *hasta bandha* (hand lock) and helps engage the muscles of the arm and torso for more support. In mountain II or valley I, move through upward-facing dog as part of the flow series or sun salutations.

## Modification

If you're healing from a wrist or lower-back injury, practice cobra pose.

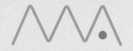

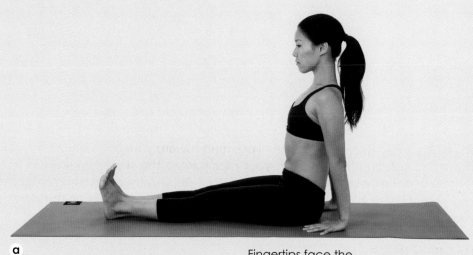

a

Fingertips face the
front of the mat

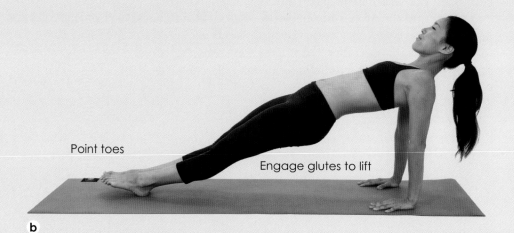

Point toes

Engage glutes to lift

b

Use incline plank pose in mountain III to stretch the front of your body and build core strength in the back of your body.

## Getting Into the Pose

From a seated position, extend your legs. Place your palms on the floor behind you with your fingertips spread and pointing toward your body (figure *a*). Press down through your hands to lift your hips toward the sky. Keeping your legs together, point your toes toward the floor. Keep the shoulders pulled down and away from the ears, keeping the back of the neck long. Avoid letting the head drop back.

## Holding the Pose

Engage your gluteal muscles and continue lifting your hips, keeping your body straight; maintain a slight bend in your elbows to avoid locking out your joints (figure *b*). For a deepening sensation, activate hasta bandha (hand lock) and squeeze the shoulder blades together.

## Modifications

For wrist injuries or discomfort, make fists for wrists with the palms facing each other. If your neck fatigues, keep the chin gently tucked in toward the chest.

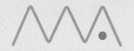

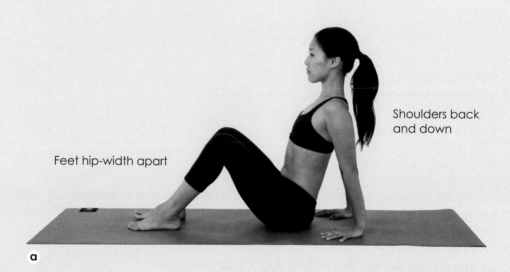

Feet hip-width apart

Shoulders back
and down

a

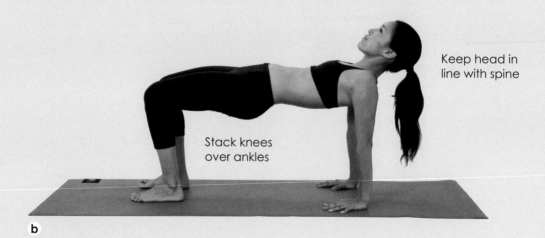

Keep head in
line with spine

Stack knees
over ankles

b

Use tabletop pose in mountain III to stretch the front of your body and build core strength in the back of your body. Because your knees are bent in table-top, this pose requires less core strength and more shoulder flexibility than what is needed for incline plank. Practice both poses to maximize the benefits.

## Getting Into the Pose

From a seated position, extend your legs. Place your palms on the floor behind you with the fingertips spread and pointing toward your body. Place the soles of your feet flat on the floor hip-width apart (figure a). Press down through your hands and feet to lift your hips toward the sky (figure b). Look straight up toward the sky without letting your head drop back.

## Holding the Pose

Engage your gluteal muscles, and continue lifting your hips, keeping your body straight. Avoid locking your elbows.

## Modifications

For wrist injuries or discomfort, make fists for wrists with the palms facing each other. If your neck fatigues, look forward rather than drop your head back.

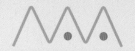

# Side Plank and Kneeling Side Plank

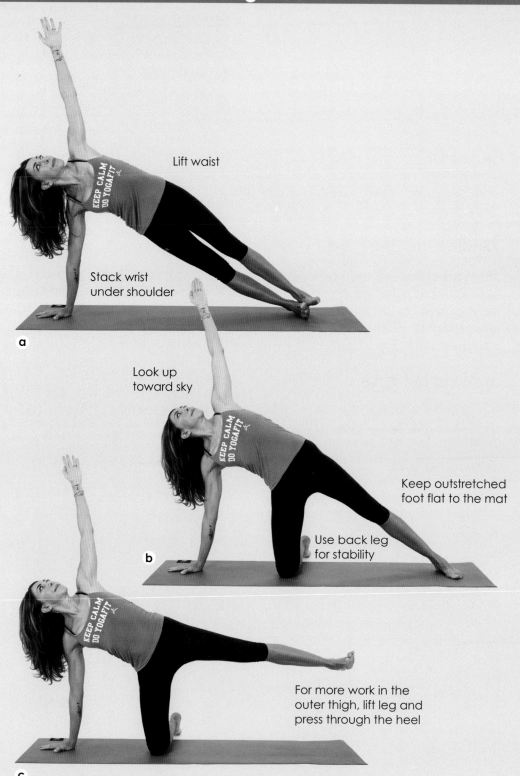

Lift waist

Stack wrist under shoulder

a

Look up toward sky

Keep outstretched foot flat to the mat

Use back leg for stability

b

For more work in the outer thigh, lift leg and press through the heel

c

Side plank and kneeling side plank target the oblique abdominal muscles, the two layers of muscle in your torso that work together to help you exhale, side bend, and twist. Practice this pose in mountain II or mountain III, using extra caution if you're healing a shoulder.

## Getting Into the Pose

**Side plank (figure *a*):** Begin in plank pose. Inhale, reaching the left arm upward and opening your torso to the left side of your mat, keeping the right wrist under the right shoulder. Roll to the edges of your feet. For a greater challenge, stack your feet and activate pada bandha through lifting the arches as if you were standing on the floor.

**Kneeling side plank (figure *b*):** From side plank pose, place your right knee below your right hip. Move your right foot slightly to the right (like a kickstand) for stability. Press your left foot into the floor, pointing your toes toward the side of your mat. Extend your left leg as you reach your left arm upward (figure c).

## Holding the Pose

For the side plank and kneeling side plank poses, lift the top side of your rib cage and waist toward the sky and press your hips forward. Look up at your top hand. Keep a slight bend in your elbow. Switch sides.

## Modifications

If you're a beginner, practice the kneeling side plank. Use extra caution if you're healing a shoulder. For wrist injuries or discomfort, make a fist instead of placing your hand flat on the floor or place the forearm on the floor with elbow stacked under the shoulder (full plank only). For knee pain or injuries, use caution and place a kneepad on the mat for comfort.

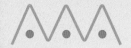

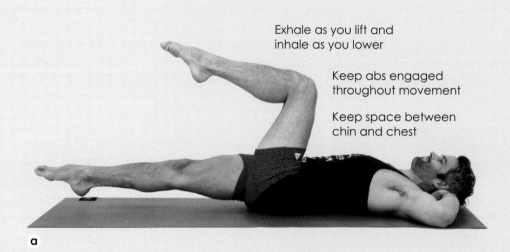

Exhale as you lift and inhale as you lower

Keep abs engaged throughout movement

Keep space between chin and chest

a

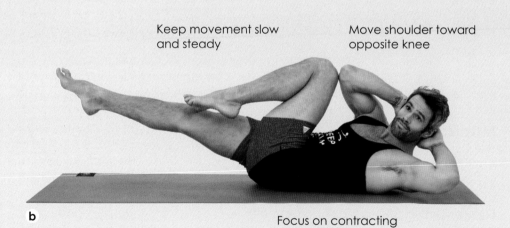

Keep movement slow and steady

Move shoulder toward opposite knee

b

Focus on contracting your obliques

Abdominal exercises isolate and strengthen the muscles in your abdomen. Because you do them on your back, you work against gravity to lift your body away from the floor, building strength and endurance. Be sure to release slowly back down to the floor instead of dropping quickly to the floor. Applying equal effort in both directions and working in pace with your breath allow you to work the muscles without the benefit of momentum, essentially for twice the strength.

When doing abdominal exercises, keep space between your chin and chest to isolate your abdominal muscles and avoid pulling on your neck. Press your lower back to the ground, keeping your stomach firm and flat. Keep your elbows back with fingers interlaced to support your head (thumbs along your neck or jaw). Exhale as you lift; inhale as you release.

In mountain I, flow abdominal exercises with your breath for muscular endurance and heat. In mountains II or III, flow with your breath or else hold and breathe three to five breaths to increase muscular strength.

## Getting Into the Pose

**Abdominal curl:** Start on your back with your feet flat on the floor and knees up. Place your hands behind your head with your fingers interlaced. As you exhale, slowly lift your head, neck, and shoulders away from the floor. Inhaling, release slowly back toward the floor without ever completely relaxing your abdomen.

**Yoga bicycle (figures *a* and *b*):** For oblique work, start on your back with your feet flat on the floor and knees up. Place your hands behind your head with the fingers interlaced. Bring one knee to your chest. Exhaling, lift your head, neck, and shoulders away from the floor. Twist, bringing the opposite elbow toward the opposite knee. Inhaling, release slowly back toward the floor without ever completely relaxing your abdomen. For an extra challenge, extend your other leg out above the floor, pushing through the heel.

## Holding the Pose

In mountains I, II, or III, flow through either exercise with your breathing or, in mountains II or III, pause at the top of the movement and breathe deeply for three to five breaths.

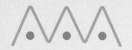

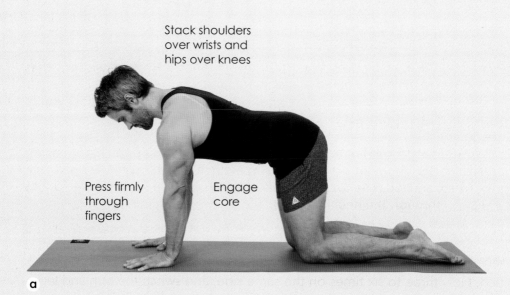

Stack shoulders over wrists and hips over knees

Press firmly through fingers

Engage core

a

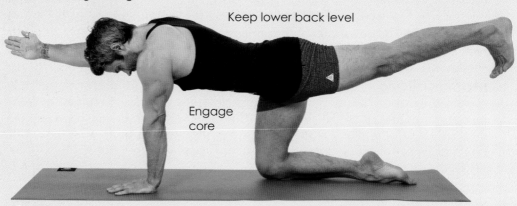

Focus on lengthening

Keep lower back level

Engage core

b

**STRENGTHENS:**
gluteal muscles • upper back •
lower back • abdominal muscles •
shoulders

Part of many fitness programs, spinal balance improves balance and increases core strength.

## Getting Into the Pose

From your hands and knees (*figure a*), extend one arm and the opposite leg parallel to the floor. Keeping a neutral spine, create a straight line with your arm, torso, and leg. The toes of the lifted leg are pointing toward the floor as you press through the heel (figure *b*).

**Powerful spinal balance:** Holding the left leg and right arm in the extended position, then using your abdominal muscles draw the elbow toward the opposite knee on the exhalation, and reach the limbs straight on the inhalation. Flow three to six times on the same side, and switch the arm and leg.

## Holding the Pose

Keep your low back level, and draw your abdominal muscles up and in. In any mountain phase, focus on reaching forward through your crown and fingers and then back through your extended foot. Remember that length is more important than lift. In mountain I, warm up your body by inhaling and lifting your opposite arm and opposite leg, releasing as you exhale and alternating sides for 5 to 10 repetitions. In mountains II or III, hold the pose for three to five breaths, and then switch sides.

## Modifications

For wrist injuries or discomfort, make fists for wrists with the palms facing each other. Or, lift just your arms or just your legs while building strength and balance. For knee pain or injuries, place a kneepad on the mat.

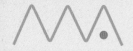

# Boat

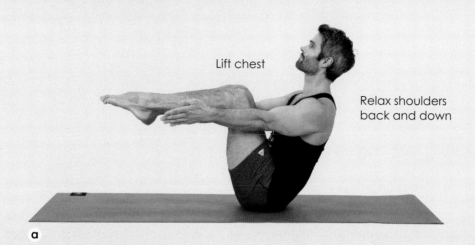

Lift chest

Relax shoulders back and down

a

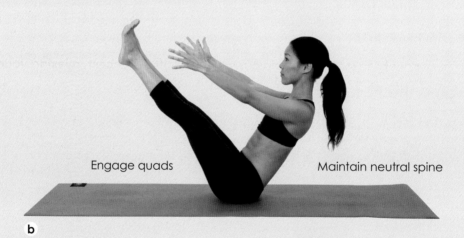

Engage quads

Maintain neutral spine

b

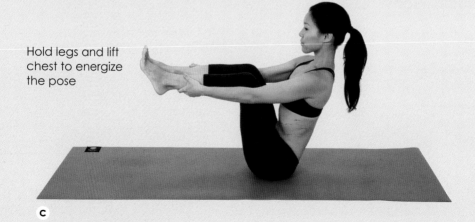

Hold legs and lift chest to energize the pose

c

Use boat pose in mountain III to strengthen your core and improve your balance. Practice boat pose after seated forward fold to assist you in maintaining a neutral spine by lengthening your back and hamstrings.

## Getting Into the Pose

Sitting tall on the floor, bend your knees and hold on to your hamstrings. Slowly lift one foot at a time away from the floor, keeping your back long. Reach forward with your arms as you balance on your sit bones (ischial tuberosities; figure a). For a greater challenge, straighten your legs and reach forward without rounding your back (figure b).

## Holding the Pose

Focus on your breath to lengthen your spine and lift your chest, relaxing your shoulders back and down (figure c).

## Modification

If you're a beginner or if you have back injuries, keep your feet on the floor and continue holding on to your hamstrings.

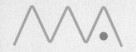

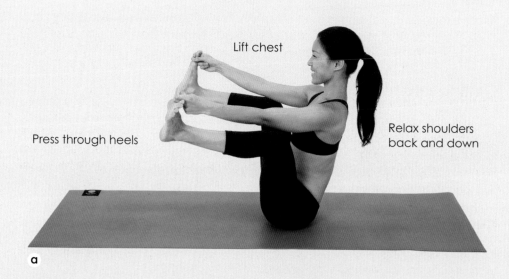

Lift chest

Press through heels

Relax shoulders back and down

a

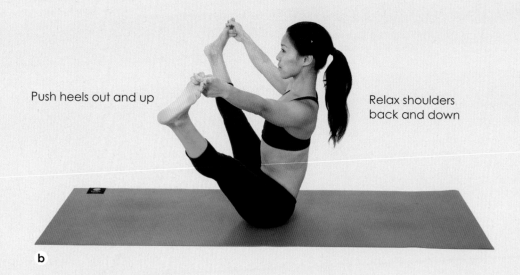

Push heels out and up

Relax shoulders back and down

b

STRENGTHENS:
upper back • biceps
STRETCHES:
hamstrings • hip adductors

This variation of boat pose focuses less on strength and more on stretching the legs. Use boat and big-toe wide boat poses in mountain III for a well-rounded practice.

## Getting Into the Pose

From boat pose, bend your knees slightly and balance on your sit bones (figure a). Loop your middle and index fingers around your big toes, inhale, and press through your heels to straighten your legs, keeping the back straight, as far as you feel comfortable.

## Holding the Pose

Pull your feet back and lift your chest up and forward, finding a point of balance (figure b). Release your feet before coming down.

## Modification

If you have tight hamstrings or difficulty balancing, keep your knees bent.

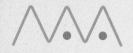

## Crow

Inhale and expand the back

Exhale and draw
navel to spine

Squeeze inner
thighs on triceps

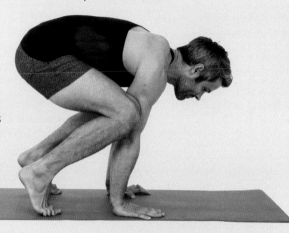

a

Glide forward with core
strongly engaged, and
as feet lift off, gently
tuck them up

Enjoy the flight with
deep, smooth breaths

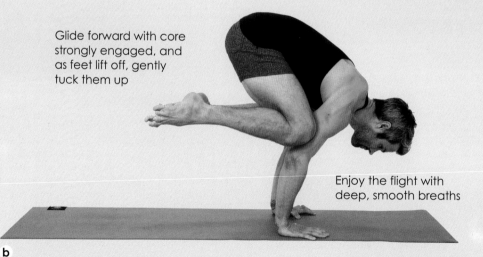

b

The following arm balances are great postures for building strength in the core muscles as well as the upper body. Practice plank and crocodile first to build a good foundation for the shoulders and the core. Arm balances can be inserted when the body is thoroughly warmed up at the end of mountain II or in mountain III if you are starting from a seated position.

This pose is nice at the end of mountain II and then followed by standing balance postures.

## Getting Into the Pose

From forward fold, position the feet slightly wider than the hips and bend the knees, placing the palms flat on the floor in starfish hands slightly in front of the shoulders. Drop the tailbone below the hips (lifting the heels as needed; figure a). Squeeze the inner thighs onto the triceps as you shift your weight smoothly onto the hands, and firmly contract the abdominal muscles by pulling the navel center toward the spine, allowing the entire back to round (figure b). Keep the gaze forward as you glide onto the hands with the elbows bending to less than 90 degrees (crocodile arms). The toes may still be resting on the floor or tucked up under the hips.

## Holding the Pose

Let the feet gently lift on their own as you focus on creating more lift through the center of the body by squeezing the inner thighs onto the arms. Breathe into the space in the back, and keep a strong contraction through the abdominal muscles. Hold for three to five breaths, and then gently glide back and rest the feet on the mat.

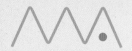

# Elephant Pose and Eight-Angle Pose

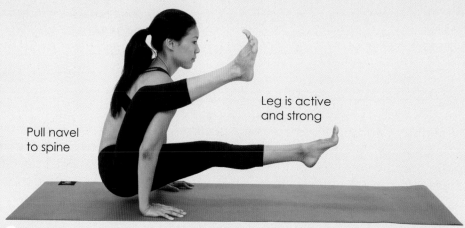

Leg is active and strong

Pull navel to spine

**a**

Push strongly into the hands

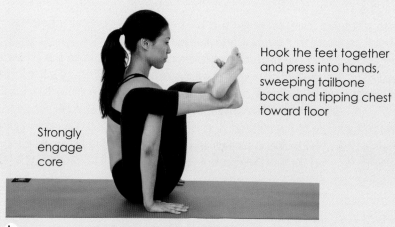

Hook the feet together and press into hands, sweeping tailbone back and tipping chest toward floor

Strongly engage core

**b**

Press firmly into the length of the fingers and thumb

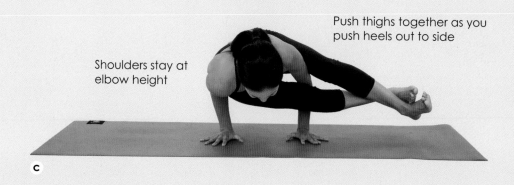

Push thighs together as you push heels out to side

Shoulders stay at elbow height

**c**

These poses are good poses to practice in mountain III after frog pose or seated butterfly. Move slowly into these poses, being mindful not to force any position before you are ready. They require a degree of hip opening, which will come gradually.

## Getting Into the Pose

From a seated position, bend your right knee while holding your right foot with the left hand. Guide your right elbow under the right thigh, placing the right palm on the floor by the hip and contracting your abdominal muscles to flex the spine (figure *a*). Place the left foot on top of the right ankle, and push through both heels to flex the feet. Placing the left palm by the left hip, press firmly down through both hands as you pull the navel toward the spine strongly and sweep the tail bone back and up (figure *b*). For more challenge, leave the left leg straight (the elephant's trunk), and contract the quadriceps as you press into the hands to lift. Hold for 5 to 10 breaths and switch sides.

From figure *a* you can progress into eight-angle pose by tipping forward once you have lifted the body off the floor, squeezing the inner thighs together, and contracting the quadriceps to extend the knees (figure *c*). Hold for 5 to 10 breaths, and switch sides.

## Holding the Pose

Keep a strong focus on the abdominal muscles in order to create lift in the pose, and keep the breath slow and deep.

# C H A P T E R 6

# Standing and Balance Poses

Most of the YogaFit standing poses are done in mountain II. They serve to increase strength and endurance (because you hold them longer) as well as increase flexibility and mobility as you continue to flow between poses. The idea that yoga is focused entirely, or primarily, on improving flexibility is a misconception. Although yoga does work to lengthen muscles and release tightness in the fascia, a fundamental intention of yoga involves balance. In both standing poses and balance poses you must be firmly grounded to enable yourself to flow easily into and out of the poses. This grounding requires a balance of stability and mobility. Proper alignment and breathing are keys to creating both stability and mobility in the flowing practice of YogaFit.

Chapter 1 introduced you to the koshas (layers of being). You can expand your thinking about balance to include the various layers of the body. Physically you can think in terms of muscles and fascia and movement of the joints. Energetically, you can think of the subtle body or the life-force energy called prana. The energy body includes the prana and your chakras (wheels) of energy. Each chakra is associated with one of the nerve plexuses that comes out of the spine and correlates with the organs and glands for that region of the body. (For detailed information on chakras, see appendix A.) Stuck energy in a particular chakra results in an imbalance in the organs and glands affected. Stiffness of the physical body can be the result of blocked prana energy, or it can create energy blockages. Each pose can help address imbalances in one or more of the chakras. For example, standing poses help balance the first chakra by helping to create a stronger foundation, while balance poses help to balance the sixth chakra by helping to increase focus.

Daily habits contribute to imbalances in the body both energetically and physically. Even being left- or right-handed (or footed) contributes to imbalance. People favor one side of the body to do everything—talking on the phone, carrying a child on one hip, swinging a golf club. Depending on work or play, people tend to favor certain positions as well. Cyclists spend hours each week crouched forward in their seat, whereas others stand all day behind a cash register, often with their weight shifted to one leg. Eventually, this kind of unconscious favoritism leads to imbalance and shows up in the form of tension headaches, minor injuries, or chronic pain. The good news is that it's never too late to get back into proper alignment. A YogaFit workout stretches and strengthens on many planes and helps bring the body back into alignment. Yoga helps to strengthen and lengthen muscle and connective tissue as well as increase the range of motion of the joints.

Most people spend a lot of time on their feet, but rarely do they stand at attention. Yoga teaches you to turn your awareness away from distractions and toward what's going on in your body. In this chapter you'll have the opportunity to recognize where you need to focus your efforts and then to patiently and persistently do the work of building strength, endurance, and flexibility as needed.

**Yoga teaches that when your body is balanced, your mind is balanced. When you feel good physically, you have more positive energy and fewer distractions. But to arrive at this point, you have to slow down and enjoy the process.**

## Standing Poses

The standing poses are used in mountains I and II (warm-up and work phases). This chapter explores these standing poses:

- Mountain
- Moonflowers
- Sunflowers
- Sun pose
- Standing lateral flexion
- Warrior I
- Warrior II
- Reverse warrior

- Triangle and extended triangle
- Side angle and extended side angle
- Bound side angle and bound triangle
- Chair and balance chair
- Prayer squat
- Warrior III
- Standing splits
- Balancing half moon

Remember that mountain I poses move with the breath. For every inhalation, you move in one direction; for every exhalation, you move in the opposite direction. Many mountain I poses can also be used in mountain II. In this case, instead of flowing with the breath, you hold the pose for three to five breaths (and, if appropriate, switch sides and repeat).

**In every standing pose you begin by bringing your awareness to your feet (SPA 1). Rather than just standing on the surface of the earth, you establish a base—the foundation on which you create all other actions in the pose. By standing with your feet hip-width apart and pressing down equally through the four corners (heels and balls) of your feet and then drawing up the arches, you activate the muscles of your legs and hips. This action engages your core, gives you stability, and lets you move into another pose when you're ready. It is helpful to practice the poses barefoot. It keeps your feet strong, flexible, and healthy, preventing problems in your ankles, knees, hips, and other areas.**

Many of the standing poses are included only in mountain II because they involve deeper stretches and greater strength. In such poses, the real work of realigning takes place. Standing yoga poses, such as the ones in this chapter, significantly increase bone density, which helps prevent osteoporosis. Men and women alike need to increase bone density as they age, and weight-bearing activities such as yoga offer excellent protection.

When practicing the standing poses, remember to do the following:

- Hold for three to five breaths.
- Practice the seven principles of alignment (SPA; see chapter 2).
- Focus on the part of your body in which you feel the most sensation.
- Listen to your breath, and let it be your guide in your practice. If it becomes rapid or shallow, rest or move to another pose; if it is long and deep, stay a little longer.

## Standing Balance Poses

These poses are the standing balance poses:

- Tree
- Eagle
- Standing balance pigeon
- Dancer
- Standing big toe hold
- Bird of paradise

The standing balance poses are done in valley II, before you come down to the floor. Although many of the standing poses in yoga require balance, these poses are done on one foot to command awareness and to identify differences between left and right.

Note that warrior III, standing splits, and balancing half moon, listed in the standing poses section, are also standing balance poses; however, because in each of them the head is not above the heart (necessary to equalize blood pressure), they are not technically considered valley II poses. That said, they can be paired with tree, eagle, standing balance pigeon, or dancer because they provide all other benefits of balance work. See notes in the warrior III, standing splits, and balancing half moon poses on how to do these poses safely in valley II.

When practicing the standing balance poses, remember to do the following:

- Practice SPA.
- Hold for 5 to 10 breaths on each side to equalize your blood pressure and improve concentration.
- Be aware of how your body feels.
- Find a focal point on the wall or floor in front of you.
- Focus on your breath. A tendency in standing balance work is to hold your breath, but if you focus on breathing the balance will come more easily.
- Relax. While working to build strength in these postures, trying too hard sometimes thwarts your efforts.

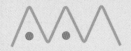

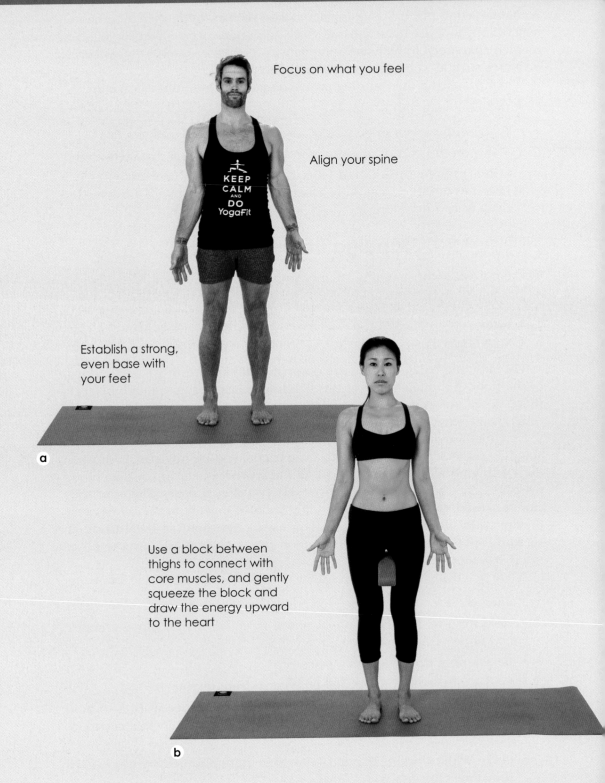

Focus on what you feel

Align your spine

Establish a strong, even base with your feet

a

Use a block between thighs to connect with core muscles, and gently squeeze the block and draw the energy upward to the heart

b

Mountain pose is often where you begin your practice, with 3 to 5 minutes of three-part breath or relaxation breath. With your eyes open or closed, this is also a strong, steady place you can come back to at any time during your practice to become aware of how your body feels and determine if you should work harder or perhaps take a step back. Just as no two mountains are alike, no two bodies are alike. Use this pose whenever necessary to appreciate your uniqueness.

## Getting Into the Pose

Stand tall at the top of your mat with your arms at your sides and feet hip-width apart. Slightly bend your knees, and press down through your feet. Reach downward through your fingers to relax your shoulders away from your ears. Lift your chest slightly, then engage your core by firmly pressing through the four corners of the feet, lifting the arches (figure a). Feel the muscle activity of the legs, draw that energy up into the torso, and pull the pelvic floor muscles up toward the heart. It may be helpful to practice mountain pose with a block between the upper thighs in order to connect with the core muscles (figure b). Remember that because muscles are connected by fascia, when you gently contract the inner thigh muscles, the pelvic floor muscles are also activated.

## Holding the Pose

Breathe deeply into your rib cage and chest, relax your shoulders and, if you like, close your eyes.

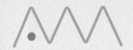

# Moonflowers

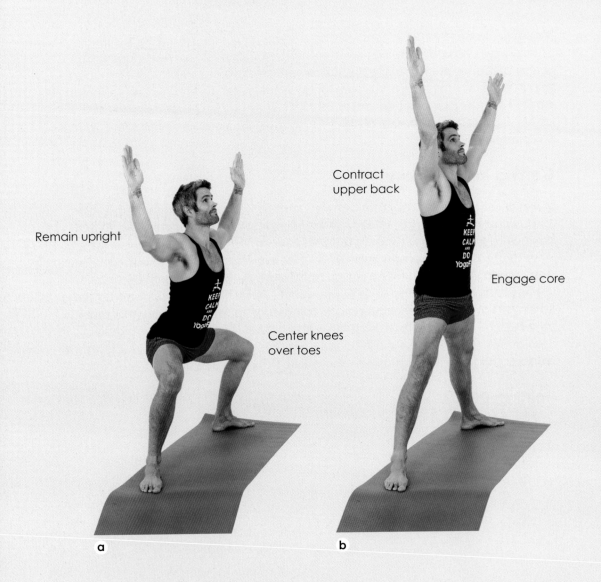

Remain upright

Center knees
over toes

Contract
upper back

Engage core

a                    b

Moonflowers is a mountain I pose. Match the pace of your movement to the pace of your breath. In YogaFit you add flowing moonflowers and sunflowers to gently begin to open the hips.

## Getting Into the Pose

Step back to face the long edge of your mat. Open your thighs, and turn your toes out and heels in for a squat. Stack your knees directly over your ankles. Bend your elbows, and place them aligned with your shoulders as you point your knees straight out over your toes (figure a). Inhale as you straighten your arms (palms forward) and legs (figure b); exhale as you come back to the starting position, drawing energy down and in. Continue to move through a comfortable range of motion as your body warms up. When ready, transition into sunflowers or another mountain I pose.

## Modification

If you have knee concerns, come only to a comfortable place in the squat, pointing your knees over the centers of your feet.

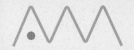

## Sunflowers

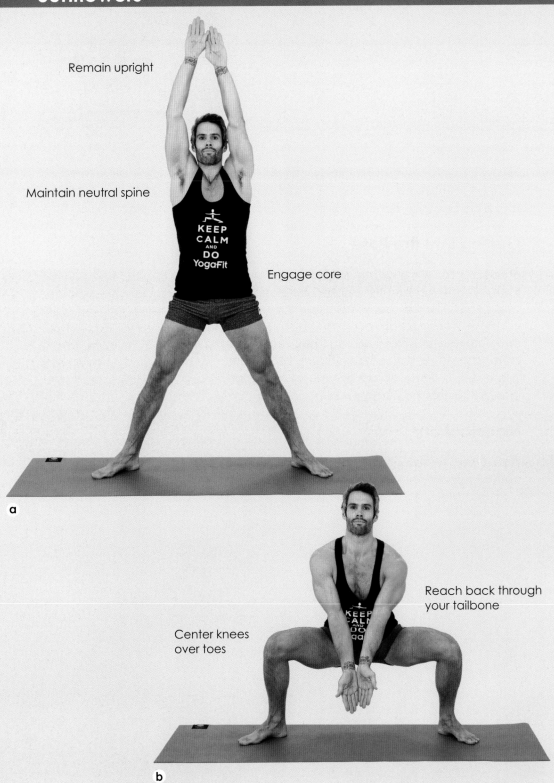

Remain upright

Maintain neutral spine

Engage core

a

Reach back through
your tailbone

Center knees
over toes

b

Sunflowers builds on moonflowers in mountain I. It works large muscle groups to build heat and moves the joints through a comfortable range of motion. Both poses prepare your body for more work and deeper stretches.

## Getting Into the Pose

Step back to face the long edge of your mat. As in moonflowers, open your thighs and turn your toes out and heels in for a squat. Bend your elbows, and place them next to your waist; point your knees straight out over your toes. Inhale as the arms move overhead (figure a); exhale as you hinge forward from the hips, reaching your tailbone back and keeping a neutral spine, sweeping your arms toward the floor (figure b). Inhaling, move back to the starting position. Continue to move through a comfortable range of motion as your body warms up.

## Modifications

If you have knee concerns, come only to a comfortable place in the squat, pointing your knees over the centers of your feet. For less intensity or shoulder concerns, place your hands on your thighs.

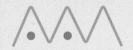

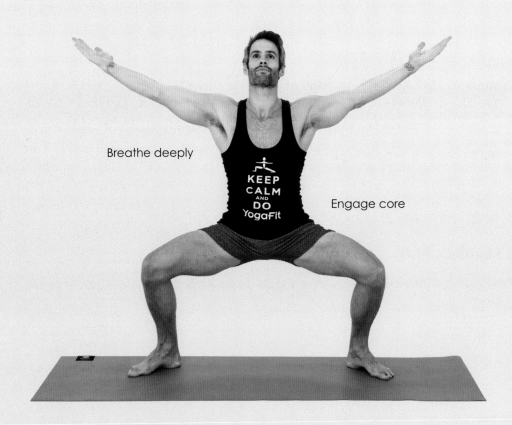

Breathe deeply

Engage core

Sun pose is a terrific mountain II pose for strengthening and toning many muscles in your legs and hips. Breathe deeply to maximize the benefits. Sun pose is also a mountain I pose.

## Getting Into the Pose

Step back to face the long edge of your mat. Open your thighs, and turn your toes out and heels in for a squat. Extend your arms, palms facing up. Slowly sink your hips, and hold. Squeeze your inner thighs to come back up.

## Holding the Pose

Press through the four corners of your feet, and squeeze the outer thighs to enhance the stretch of the inner thighs. Lift the heart, and relax the shoulders down as you reach out through the fingers.

## Modification

If you have shoulder concerns, rest your hands on your hips or thighs.

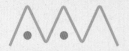

## Standing Lateral Flexion

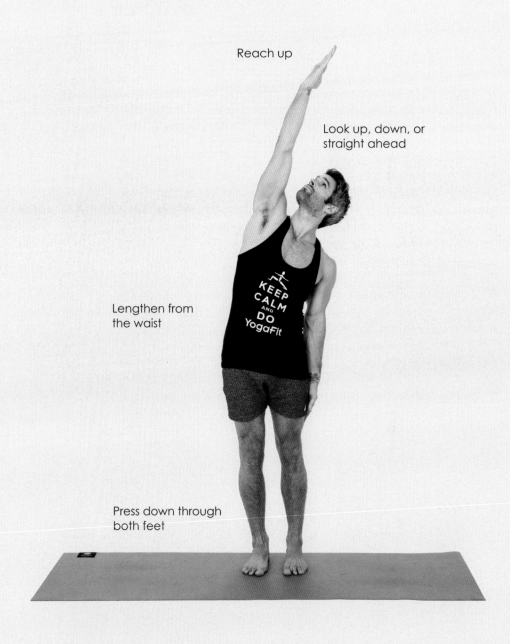

Reach up

Look up, down, or straight ahead

Lengthen from the waist

Press down through both feet

Practice this pose between standing poses to stretch and strengthen your torso. Move side to side with your breath in mountain I, or hold for three to five breaths on each side in mountain II.

## Getting Into the Pose

Lift your arms over your head. Create dynamic tension by lifting your upper body and pressing down through your feet. Slide one hand down the outer thigh, and reach the other hand toward the sky. Gently lean to the side without dropping your chest.

## Holding the Pose

In mountain II, breathe into your sides, rib cage, waist, and chest. Keep your head in line with your spine. Don't let your upper body fall forward. Come up, and switch sides.

## Modification

For more low-back support, place your lower hand on your hip.

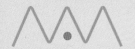

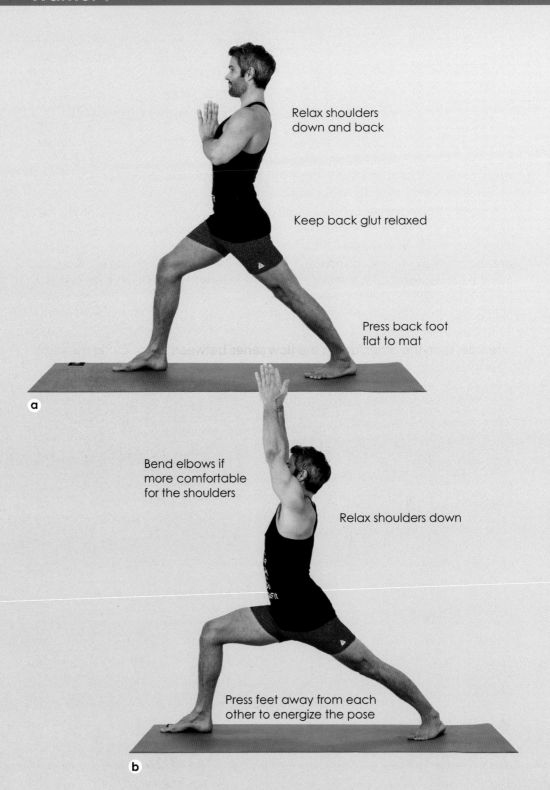

Relax shoulders down and back

Keep back glut relaxed

Press back foot flat to mat

a

Bend elbows if more comfortable for the shoulders

Relax shoulders down

Press feet away from each other to energize the pose

b

This pose is part of the warrior series. Benefits include increased physical and mental strength, enhanced power, and determination. This mountain II pose is often repeated several times in a session followed by other standing mountain II poses.

The warrior poses—warrior I, warrior II, reverse warrior, and warrior III (discussed later in the chapter)—are primarily focused on building heat and strength. When you hold these challenging standing positions steady and breathe deeply, you also increase your ability to deal with stress. Keep in mind that aggression, however, saps your strength: A peaceful warrior is a powerful warrior.

Try the warrior poses in a sequence with other standing mountain II poses, such as warrior I, warrior II, reverse warrior, or triangle. Do the series first on one side, then the other, doing the flow series between them. Or do the same pose once on each side before moving on.

Note: YogaFit teaches two variations of warrior I to avoid creating tension and pain in the low back and hip. Use a short stance (figure a) for moving into other forward facing poses (i.e., pyramid) and a long stance (figure b) if you are moving into open-hip stances (i.e., warrior II). In the long-stance warrior I, instead of squaring the hips forward, you will feel a twist in the torso as you move toward squaring your shoulders forward.

## Getting Into the Pose

From mountain pose, step back into a short stance and align your heels. Bend your front knee, stacking it over your ankle. Straighten your back leg, turning your toes slightly forward. Square your hips or shoulders with the front of your mat (depending on your stance). Raise your arms to the sky.

## Holding the Pose

Continue to press the outer edge of your back foot into the mat. Open your hands and spread your fingers wide. Relax your shoulders down. Engage your abdominals as you lift up with your upper body and sink into your forward leg. Keep your forward knee over your ankle.

## Modifications

To decrease the intensity, slightly straighten your forward leg, shorten your stance, or both. For shoulder discomfort, bring the palms of your hands together at the center of your chest (prayer position).

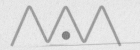

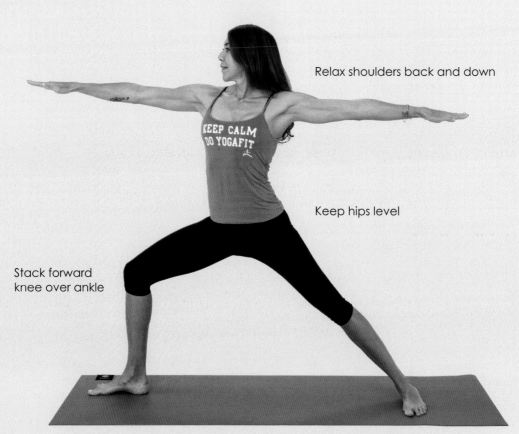

Relax shoulders back and down

Keep hips level

Stack forward
knee over ankle

Point back toes
toward long
edge of mat

In mountain II, warrior II follows warrior I pose. Here, for improved strength, focus, and discipline, emphasize moving energy outward while turning your awareness inward. (See the discussion in the warrior I pose for more information on the benefits of the warrior poses.)

## Getting Into the Pose

From a long-stance warrior I pose, keep your heels aligned as you open your hips and shoulders to the long edge of your mat. Lower your arms parallel to the floor, reaching out in opposite directions through your fingers. Keep your front knee bent and hips level. Look over your front hand.

## Holding the Pose

Press through the feet, lifting the arches (activating pada bandha) to create the lift in your upper body. Keep the front knee stacked over the front ankle, and reach the arms in opposite directions. Engage the abdominal muscles, and relax your shoulders back and down. If you feel fatigued, focus on your hands to boost your energy. Open your palms and spread your fingers wide to bring the entire pose to life.

## Modifications

To decrease the intensity, slightly straighten the forward leg, shorten your stance, or do both. For shoulder discomfort, bring your palms together in prayer position. For low-back discomfort, shorten the stance and engage the abdominal muscles by drawing the abs up toward the heart.

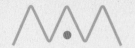

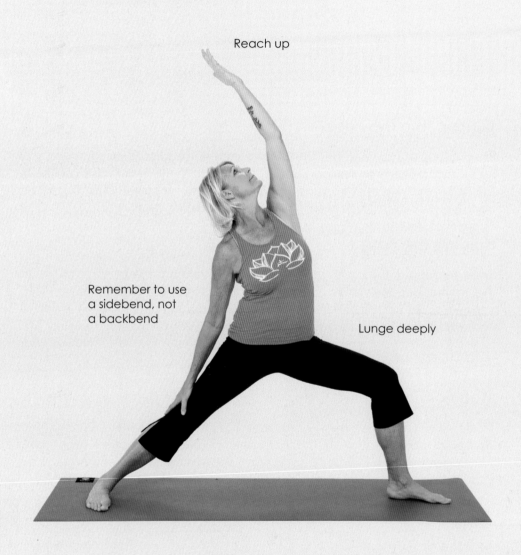

Reach up

Remember to use
a sidebend, not
a backbend

Lunge deeply

Practice reverse warrior in mountain II to stretch and strengthen your upper and lower body. (See pose titled Warrior I to learn the benefits of the warrior poses.)

## Getting Into the Pose

From warrior II, keep your front knee bent and lift your forward arm toward the sky. Turn your forward palm up and over your head, toward the back of your mat. Rest your back hand lightly on your back leg. Use core strength to support a gentle side bend.

## Holding the Pose

Press through the feet, feeling the strength in your lower body while lifting up and out of your waist. Watch your knee-to-ankle alignment on your forward leg. Switch sides.

## Modifications

To decrease intensity, slightly straighten your forward leg or shorten your stance, or do both. For shoulder discomfort, bring your palms together in prayer position.

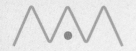

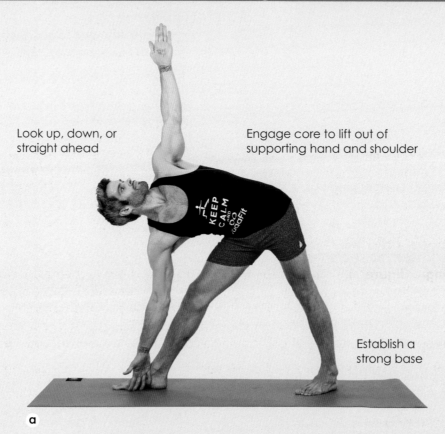

Look up, down, or straight ahead

Engage core to lift out of supporting hand and shoulder

Establish a strong base

a

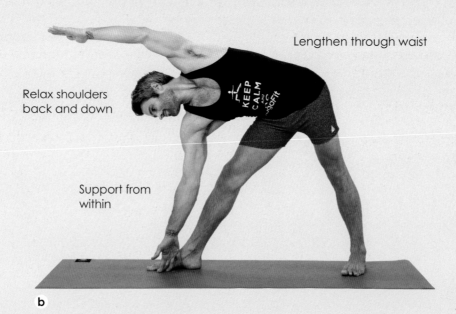

Lengthen through waist

Relax shoulders back and down

Support from within

b

Triangle pose and extended triangle pose represent a strong mental and physical foundation formed by the two bottom points of the triangle. From here, you can begin looking up to explore the third point—the spiritual. Practice these poses within the mountain II portion of your workout.

## Getting Into the Pose

**Triangle (figure *a*):** From warrior II or side angle pose, straighten your front leg. Moving from the front hip, tilt the upper body toward the front of your mat while maintaining a strong core and neutral spine, reaching your hand toward your shin or ankle. Lift your back arm to the sky, opening your chest. Look up, down, or straight ahead, finding a comfortable position for your neck.

**Extended triangle (figure *b*):** For an added challenge, from triangle pose, drop your top arm over your ear and roll your chest toward the sky.

## Holding the Pose

Press your feet away from each other, keeping a slight bend in your forward knee. Your nose stays over your leg, not in front of it. Pressing into the feet will create dynamic tension through the legs and gluteal muscles to support the pose. Breathe length into your spine, allowing your inner strength to fuel your outer strength. Switch sides.

## Modification

If your hamstrings or inner thighs are tight, place your lower hand on a block or your thigh.

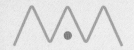

# Side Angle and Extended Side Angle

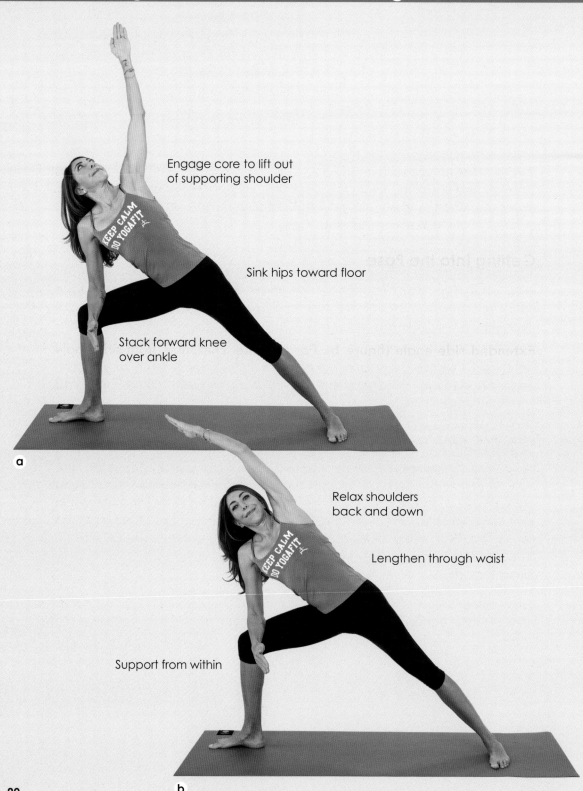

Engage core to lift out
of supporting shoulder

Sink hips toward floor

Stack forward knee
over ankle

a

Relax shoulders
back and down

Lengthen through waist

Support from within

b

Practice side angle and extended side angle pose within mountain II to build strength and flexibility in your legs and hips. Your oblique abdominal muscles also get a great workout as you lengthen your spine over your forward leg and roll your chest toward the sky.

## Getting Into the Pose

**Side angle (figure *a*):** From a warrior stance, bend your front knee and place your forearm on your thigh, or place your hand in front of your leg on the floor. Reach your top arm to the sky.

**Extended side angle (figure *b*):** For a greater challenge, from side angle pose, reach your top arm over your head until your biceps is over your ear, palm facing down. Reach forward through your fingertips as you push into your back foot.

## Holding the Pose

In either pose, rotate your chest toward the sky and press your hand into the earth. If your forearm is resting on the thigh, remember not to lean into the arm but rather keep the core active. Press into the feet to activate dynamic tension in the legs and core while lowering your hips. With every inhalation, lengthen your spine. With every exhalation, press further into the feet. Switch sides.

## Modification

For either version of the pose, place your bottom hand on a block to help lift and support your torso as you build core strength.

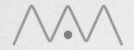

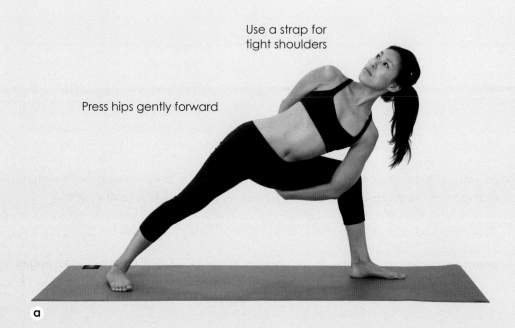

Use a strap for tight shoulders

Press hips gently forward

a

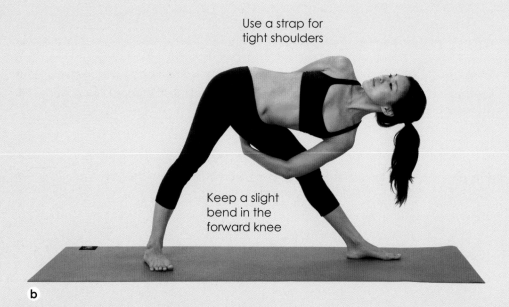

Use a strap for tight shoulders

Keep a slight bend in the forward knee

b

Binding any yoga pose should allow for more freedom, not tie you in knots. Practice bound triangle pose and bound side angle pose within mountain II for more heat, strength through your quadriceps and waist, and openness through your chest and shoulders. You will know you are ready to progress to this pose when you are no longer relying on the bottom arm to prop up the extended side angle pose, meaning the support is truly coming from within. Remember, as intensity increases, so does your need to breathe deeply.

## Getting Into the Pose

**Bound side angle (figure *a*):** From side angle pose or extended side angle pose, bring your forward hand inside your front foot. Reach behind your back with your top hand as you reach beneath your forward leg with your bottom hand, clasping them together. Lean back. Press into your feet while lowering your hips toward the floor, and roll your chest toward the sky.

**Bound triangle (figure *b*):** From bound side angle pose, slowly straighten your forward leg, keeping a microbend in your knee.

## Holding the Pose

Keep your back foot planted. Look up, down or forward, focusing on your breath. Make sure that the torso is stacked over the front thigh, and rotate the chest upward. Switch sides.

## Modification

If unable to clasp your hands, use a hand towel or strap. Begin by placing the strap in your top hand and reaching for it from below.

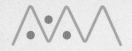

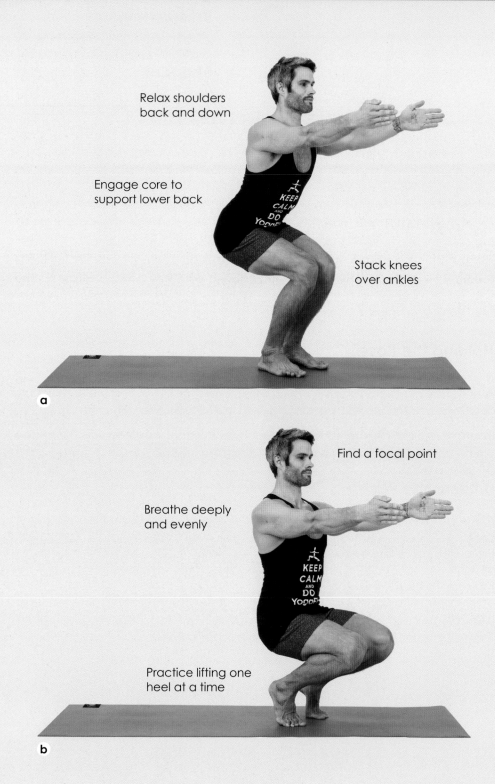

Relax shoulders
back and down

Engage core to
support lower back

Stack knees
over ankles

a

Find a focal point

Breathe deeply
and evenly

Practice lifting one
heel at a time

b

In mountain I, you move in and out of chair pose with every breath to warm up. In mountain II, you hold chair pose or balance chair pose to increase stability, power, and strength in your lower body. Chair pose is also included in sun salutations as part of valley I.

## Getting Into the Pose

**Chair (figure *a*):** Bend your knees and drop your buttocks, as if sitting in a chair.

**Balance chair (figure *b*):** From chair pose, lift your heels and balance on the balls of your feet, sitting a bit lower. Keeping your chest lifted, find a focal point and breathe. Practice lifting just one heel at a time.

## Holding the Pose

Reach back with your tailbone. Lift your chest to the sky. Lift your arms parallel to the floor, keeping the elbows slightly bent. Support your low back by engaging your core. Keep your knees behind your toes by shifting your weight to your heels (for chair pose).

## Modification

Rest your hands on your thighs for more support. For balance chair, use caution if you're healing a foot or knee injury.

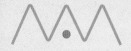

Keep head in line with spine

Press triceps into inner thigh

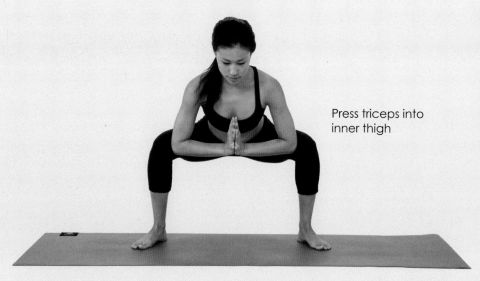

This pose helps build strength and endurance in the legs while opening the hips. A heat-building pose that can build confidence and personal power, it can be practiced in mountain II.

## Getting Into the Pose

From mountain pose, step one foot back and turn to the side, positioning the feet a little wider than hip-width apart. Slowly lower the hips to knee level, keeping the knees stacked over the ankles and keeping the spine in neutral with a strong core. You can place your hands on your thighs or bring the palms together in prayer position.

## Holding the Pose

Keep the core strong by continuing to press into the feet and lift the arches. If comfortable, lower the hips further and place the triceps against the inner thighs, pressing the arms into the legs and the legs into the arms, creating dynamic tension. You can drop lower if your knees are healthy, but be mindful to keep the knee and ankle joints aligned.

## Modifications

If you are taking care of your knees, keep the hips higher than the knees. Place the hands on the thighs for more back support.

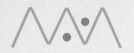

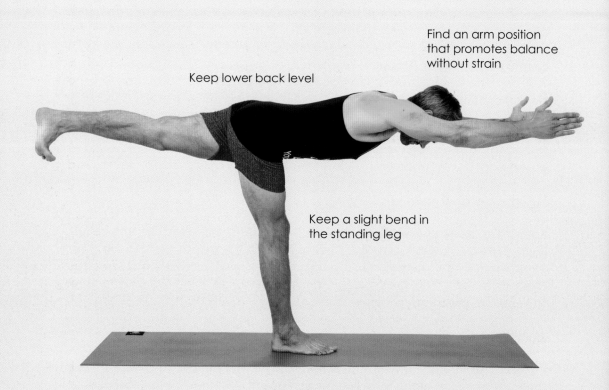

Keep lower back level

Find an arm position that promotes balance without strain

Keep a slight bend in the standing leg

**STRENGTHENS:**
gluteal muscles • upper back •
lower back • abdominal muscles •
concentration

**STRETCHES:**
hamstrings

Warrior III brings the strength and heat-building elements of a warrior pose into the practice of balance. (See pose earlier in this chapter titled warrior I for the benefits of the warrior poses.) You can practice this dynamic pose within mountain II or valley II. If in valley II, follow the pose with a second standing balance pose with your body upright to help regulate your blood pressure before coming to the floor for mountain III.

## Getting Into the Pose

Stand in mountain pose with your arms overhead or out to the sides. Extend one leg back, and hinge from your hips to lower your torso until both the leg and the torso are parallel to the floor.

## Holding the Pose

Lengthen in opposite directions away from your navel. Imagine pressing the lifted foot into an imaginary wall behind you to find more dynamic tension. Breathe deeply to make your body longer and lighter. Switch sides.

## Modifications

To decrease intensity, bring your arms out to the sides or rest them lightly on the standing thigh. Bend or straighten your standing leg as needed for balance.

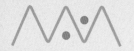

## Standing Splits

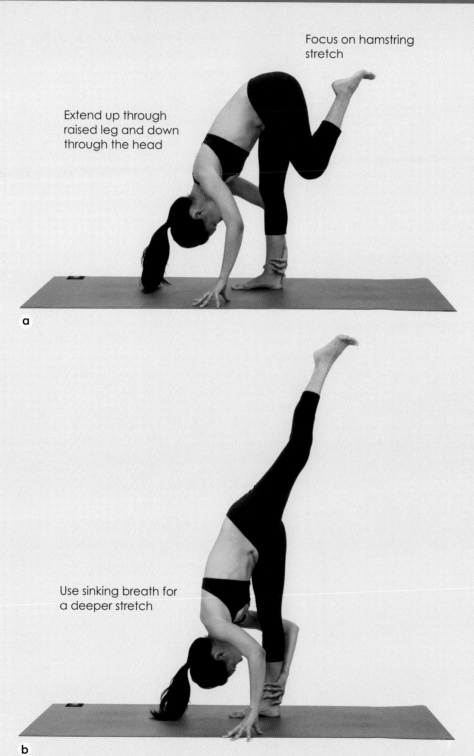

Focus on hamstring stretch

Extend up through raised leg and down through the head

**a**

Use sinking breath for a deeper stretch

**b**

Like warrior III, standing splits can be practiced within mountain II or valley II. If in valley II, follow the pose with a second standing balance pose with your body upright to help regulate your blood pressure before coming to the floor for mountain III.

## Getting Into the Pose

Place your hands on the floor, and lift one leg toward the sky while drawing your torso toward your thigh. For greater challenge, hold your standing ankle with one hand, keeping your other hand on the mat (figure *a*).

## Holding the Pose

Continue to reach up through your top leg and down through the crown of your head (figure *b*). Look at your big toe or back into your shin. Switch sides.

## Modification

If you have tight hamstrings or trouble balancing, bend your standing leg as necessary.

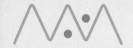

# Balancing Half Moon

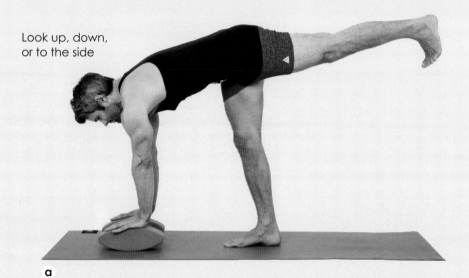

Look up, down,
or to the side

a

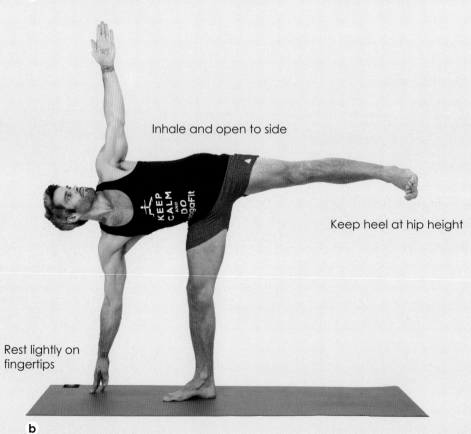

Inhale and open to side

Keep heel at hip height

Rest lightly on
fingertips

b

**STRENGTHENS:**
oblique abdominal muscles •
hip abductors • concentration
**STRETCHES:**
hamstrings

You have the additional use of your hand in this balance pose, but you experience an added challenge of holding your spine parallel (or nearly parallel) to the floor. Practice this pose near the end of mountain II or in valley II when your body is thoroughly warm. In valley II, follow this pose with an upright standing balance pose.

## Getting Into the Pose

From standing forward fold pose or pyramid pose, raise your back leg level with your hip. Place your forward fingertips on the floor or on a pair of YogaFit egg blocks directly beneath your shoulder (figure *a*). For a greater challenge, enter the balancing half moon from warrior III or standing splits, bending your standing leg as necessary for balance and control as you transition.

## Holding the Pose

When balanced, roll your chest toward the sky and extend your top arm overhead (figure *b*). Then look up to your top hand. For added challenge, keep weight out of the lower hand by pressing into the standing leg and activating your core, then imagine playing the piano with your lower hand while remaining steady and balanced. Stay focused, breathing deeply. Switch sides.

## Modifications

If your hamstrings are tight, use a block under the bottom hand. If you have shoulder instability or a rotator cuff injury, avoid leaning on the front arm, instead using more core. This pose is also beautifully supported with your back against a wall so that you can opening fully without the challenge of balancing or fear of falling.

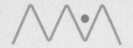

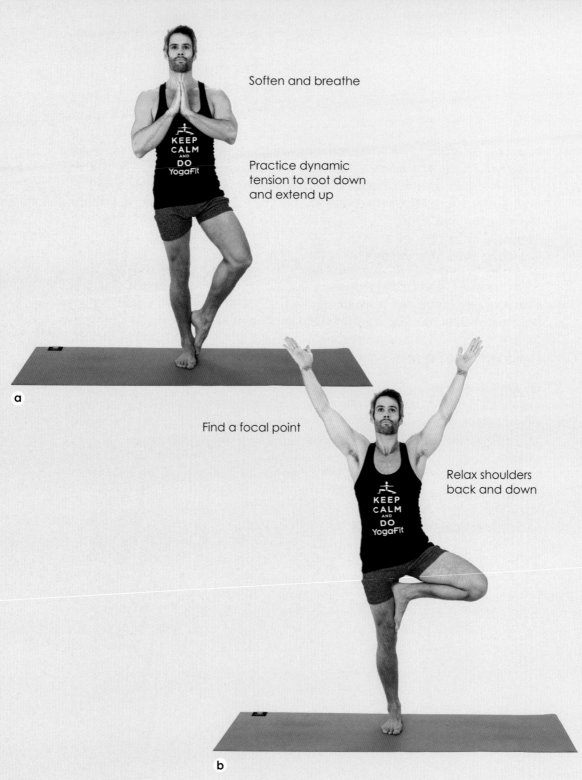

Soften and breathe

Practice dynamic tension to root down and extend up

a

Find a focal point

Relax shoulders back and down

b

**STRENGTHENS:**
  hip abductors • abdominal muscles • shoulders • concentration
**STRETCHES:**
  latissimus dorsi • hip adductors

This popular valley II pose promotes poise and calm. Visualize yourself as a tree, rooting down through your standing leg and expanding upward and outward through your arms as if they were branches. Play with your arm and foot positions until you find a steady place to hold the pose and breathe.

## Getting Into the Pose

Balance on one leg. Without using your hands, bring your opposite foot onto your standing ankle, calf, or inner thigh, avoiding the knee joint. Bring the palms together in prayer position (figure *a*). For a greater challenge, raise your arms overhead and look up (figure *b*).

## Holding the Pose

Lift up through the crown of your head while firmly rooting through your standing foot. Contract your abdominal muscles, and level your hips. Switch sides.

## Modifications

If you have difficulty balancing, place the toes of your raised leg on the mat, or stand next to a wall for support. Use caution in this pose if you have knee concerns.

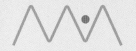

# Eagle

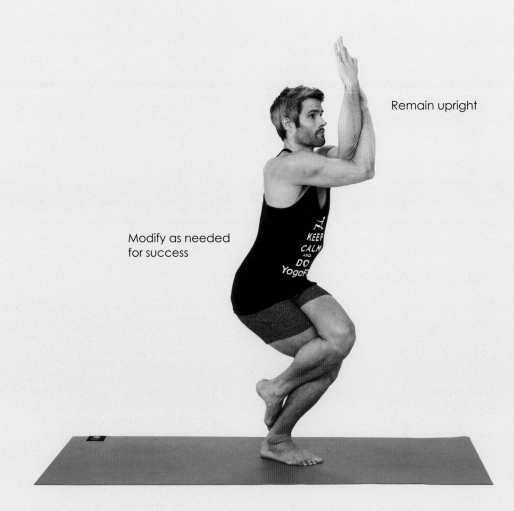

Remain upright

Modify as needed
for success

Similar to tree pose, this valley II pose works well after the body is warm to improve balance and focus.

## Getting Into the Pose

Wrap your top leg around your standing leg, squeezing the inner thighs together for more stability. Touch your toes to the mat or hook your foot behind your calf. Sit back with your hips, keeping your spine upright. Wrap your arms to touch your palms (or back of your hands) together. The top leg is the same side as the top arm.

## Holding the Pose

Stretch upward, and visualize drawing energy toward the sky as you root down through the standing foot. Contract your abdominal muscles, and keep your shoulders and tailbone low. Breathe into the space in the upper back to enhance sensation. Switch sides.

## Modifications

If you feel unstable, stand near a wall for support. If you have knee concerns, use caution in this pose.

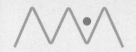

# Standing Balance Pigeon

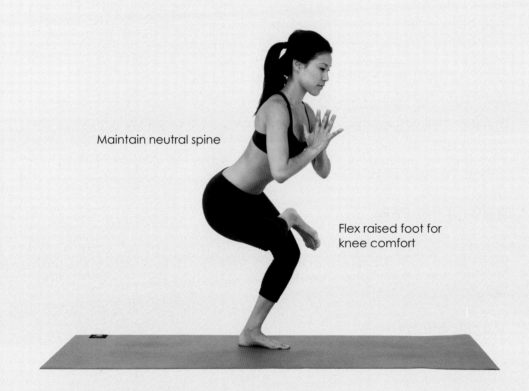

Maintain neutral spine

Flex raised foot for knee comfort

**STRENGTHENS:**
quadriceps • lower back •
concentration
**STRETCHES:**
hip adductors • hip abductors

In this valley II pose, you gain all the benefits of balancing while getting a great hip stretch. This is a favorite of walkers, runners, and bikers. Because overworked, tense muscles respond well to heat, practice this pose when your body is thoroughly warm.

## Getting Into the Pose

Begin in a chair pose (see earlier in this chapter). Shift your weight to one foot. When balanced, place your opposite ankle across your standing thigh. Press through the heel of your lifted foot, and bring your hands to your chest in prayer position.

## Holding the Pose

Find a focal point and continue lengthening your spine with every breath. Engage your abdominals to support your low back. For more sensation, lower the hips while keeping the spine in neutral and the knee of the supporting leg stacked over the ankle. Switch sides.

## Modification

If you feel unstable, stand near a wall for support.

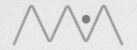

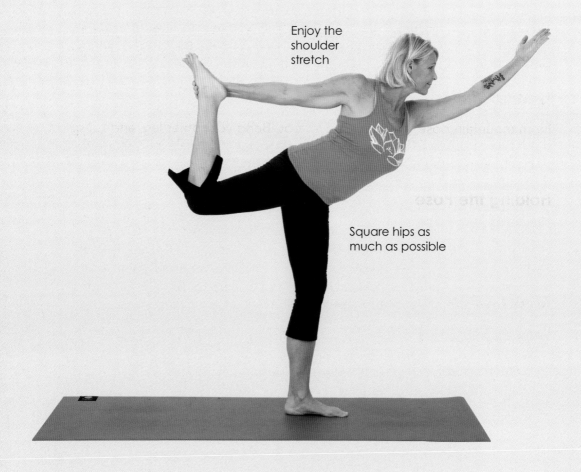

Enjoy the shoulder stretch

Square hips as much as possible

Do dancer pose in valley II. Because this pose stretches the front of your hips and opens your chest, it relieves tightness caused by long periods of sitting, walking, running, or cycling.

## Getting Into the Pose

From mountain pose, balance on one foot. Bend your other leg, and grasp the inside of your ankle with the hand on the same side, palm out. Reach the opposite arm to the sky, and slowly hinge forward.

## Holding the Pose

Continue extending in opposite directions. Pull your ankle higher as you lift your forward arm. Square your hips with the front of mat. For more backbend, lift the chest upward. Switch sides.

## Modification

If you feel unstable, place your hand on a wall in front of you for support.

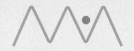

## Standing Big Toe Hold

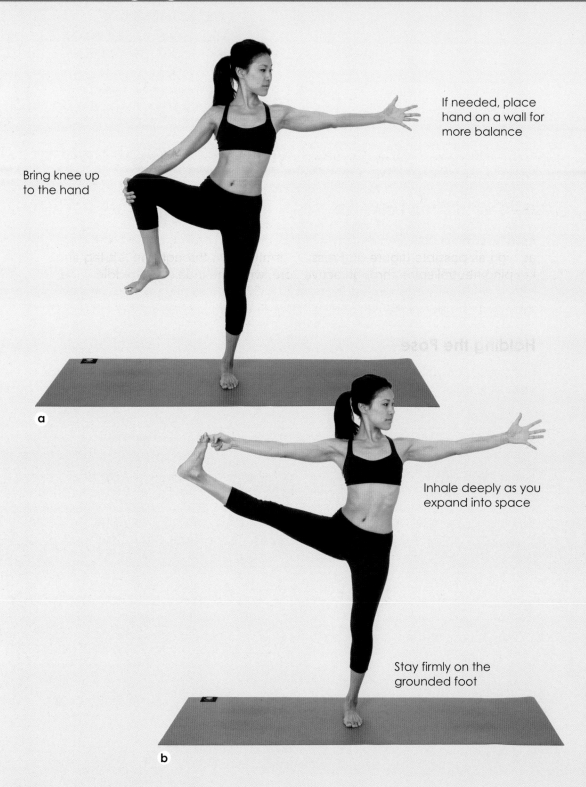

If needed, place hand on a wall for more balance

Bring knee up to the hand

**a**

Inhale deeply as you expand into space

Stay firmly on the grounded foot

**b**

Practice this pose in valley II. It provides an empowering hip opener while also working on focus and balance.

## Getting Into the Pose

From mountain pose, flex the right hip to bring the knee up toward your chest as high as possible (figure a). Pressing firmly down through the left leg and keeping neutral spine through active core, wrap the index and middle finger of the right hand around the right big toe. Either hold this position, or push through the right heel to extend the knee (figure b).

## Holding the Pose

Pressing firmly into the left foot and sweeping the left hand out to the side, lift through the chest for more opening in the chest and shoulders. Release slowly, and repeat on the other side.

## Modifications

Use a strap to hold the extended foot, or keep the foot lifted without holding on to it. If your hamstrings are tight, externally rotate the thigh.

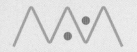

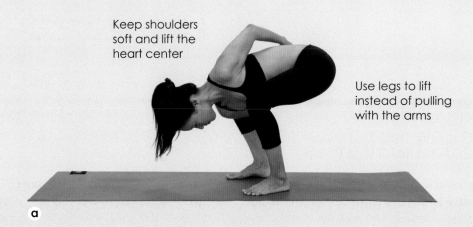

Keep shoulders soft and lift the heart center

Use legs to lift instead of pulling with the arms

a

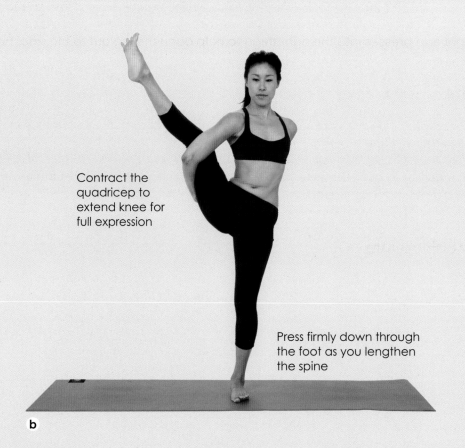

Contract the quadricep to extend knee for full expression

Press firmly down through the foot as you lengthen the spine

b

**STRENGTHENS:**
gluteal muscles • legs • shoulders • arms • core

**STRETCHES:**
shoulders • chest • hip adductors • hamstrings

Practice this pose at the end of mountain II or in valley II after a thorough warm-up of the hips.

## Getting Into the Pose

From chair pose, walk the feet a little wider than hip-width apart. Lowering the hips, bring the right upper arm inside the right leg. Reach under the leg, then wrap the left arm behind the back, finding the right hand, and clasp hands (figure *a*). Shifting weight to the left foot, begin to slowly press into the foot using the power of the legs and core to come into a standing position. The right arm presses into the right thigh to help open the leg out to the side. For increased sensation, straighten the right leg.

## Holding the Pose

Breathe fully and deeply into the lungs while lifting the chest. Pull the hands in opposite directions to create more opening in the chest and shoulders (figure *b*). Hold the position for 5 to 10 breaths, and switch sides. For more challenge you can come into this pose from bound angle pose. With the right leg forward, bring the left leg to the front of the mat and then shift weight into the left leg, following the earlier instructions.

## Modifications

Use a strap for tight shoulders and chest. You can practice this pose without binding. Keep the right triceps against the right thigh while the left hand reaches around the back and holds onto the back of the waistband.

# CHAPTER 7

# Forward and Backward Bends

How you set up your practice and move the spine affects the nervous system and thus your health. The effects may be most noticed in the case of forward bending and backbending. Generally forward bends are known to be calming and soothing, whereas backbends tend to be more stimulating and help to elevate mood. Many of the activities of daily life involve rounding forward. Think about how much time people spend driving, sitting at computers, and looking down at phones—leading to the forward-flexion lifestyle described in chapter 3. The result of this posture is tight chest muscles and shoulders and also tight hips resulting from hours of sitting. So why practice it even more on your mat? Because most of the forward bending in daily life is done through the spinal column, where you round the shoulders and bend from the waist instead of hinging from the hips with a long, straight spine. Bending the way people do many times a day compromises posture and leads to back pain and injuries. People with excessive rounding of the upper back (a postural abnormality known as excessive kyphosis) are known to live shorter life spans. You can counter this condition and improve your posture in your yoga practice. The SPA principle of hinging at the hips (see chapter 2) is specifically meant for taking care of your back. In a vinyasa practice we come into and out of forward fold many times. YogaFit teaches you to hinge at the hips and use a swan dive so that the spine stays in neutral, and you use the legs to power the movement. The more you practice hip hinging on the mat, the more likely you are to prevent back injuries both on and off your mat.

As many hours as people spend bending forward, the opposite is true of bending backward. In fact, people don't spend nearly enough time in the backbend position. It has been said that the neck was created to allow people to look up at the stars, but how often do people really do this? In this forward-bending society people rarely extend their spines in any sort of backbend to perform daily tasks, and poor postural habits are affecting their health. Slouching compresses the heart and lungs, potentially taking years off a person's life. Poor posture can also lead to chronic pain and back injuries. Improving your posture does more than improve your physical health. Posture can reflect mood. The old saying *Chin up!* suggests that sadness and defeat can cause people to slouch. Although the simple act of lifting your head and standing tall might not fix an unfortunate situation, it can certainly help you feel better. It is also known that backbending compresses your adrenal glands, located in the low back, in a way that can energize you and prepare you for action. Backbending postures are used in India to help those with heart disease. If you open the chest and shoulders, you have more space to breathe deeply, thus getting more oxygen into your body. Simply improving your posture enough to take deeper breaths can have powerful effects on your health and your mood.

> Forward bending and backward bending nourish the spine. Between each vertebra of your spine are shock absorbers called discs. The only way to keep these discs soft and supple is to manipulate them through spinal movement. A YogaFit workout ensures that you move your entire spine in every direction—forward, backward, sideways, and rotating—through a range of motion that honors your body rather than injuring it.

Pay attention to your low back. When practicing backbends, most people favor this area. Although favoring the low back may seem easier at first, in the long run it can cause pain and injury. The majority of people in the United States will at some point experience back pain. This is a shame, because many of these injuries could be avoided through a program of strengthening and stretching that focuses on movement throughout the spine, not just the low back, which is often the most flexible. When it comes to your spine in backward bends, focus on going long rather than deep. Your back will thank you.

You'll perform forward bends and backbends in mountains I, II, and III (warm-up, workout, and cool-down). Milder backbends, such as cobra pose, are safe in mountain I, but make sure your body is warm before you try the deeper backbends.

**Principles of Forward and Backward Bends**

When practicing forward and backward bends, apply these principles:

- Relax and breathe while moving into and out of the postures. In general you exhale into forward bends and inhale into backbends. Continuous breathing helps you avoid forcing yourself beyond safe ranges of motion. Breathing while holding poses helps to lengthen tight hamstrings and low-back muscles. It also relaxes you and fights the harmful effects of stress on your mind and body. Any time you're holding a forward bend, practice the sinking breath technique (see chapter 3). Focus on completing your exhalation and elongating and releasing muscles from the backs of your legs, up your spine, to even that tight place between your ears. Any time you hold a backbend, use the expanding breath technique (see chapter 3), opening with every inhalation, and holding the expansion with every exhalation. Keep your head in line with your spine, allowing it to continue the curve either forward or back.

- Perform one of the two recommended warm-ups (described in chapter 10) for at least 15 minutes before practicing deep backbends.

- As you learned in SPA 1 (see chapter 2), when practicing backbends, always begin with your base and work up. Also, be sure to engage your core to protect your back.

- Keep your knees slightly bent during all standing forward-bending poses. If you have a low-back injury or a hamstring injury, bend your knees more to shorten the hamstrings for less strain on the muscles and decreased tension on the pelvis. Whether you are sitting or standing in a forward fold, bring the belly to the thighs and lengthen the back. When you allow your pelvis to tip forward into a forward-folding pose, you put less strain on your spine and the muscles of your low back.

- Use counterposes to balance your body after deep stretches and releases, especially after vigorous backbends. Follow every backbend with a few breaths in a neutral spine position, then perform a forward bend. Or, if you're practicing backbends from the floor, such as bridge pose or wheel pose, follow the pose with bringing the knees to the chest.

- The swan dive and reverse swan dive are always used as transitions between standing forward fold and any upright standing pose (see important reminders about SPA in chapter 2).

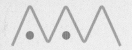

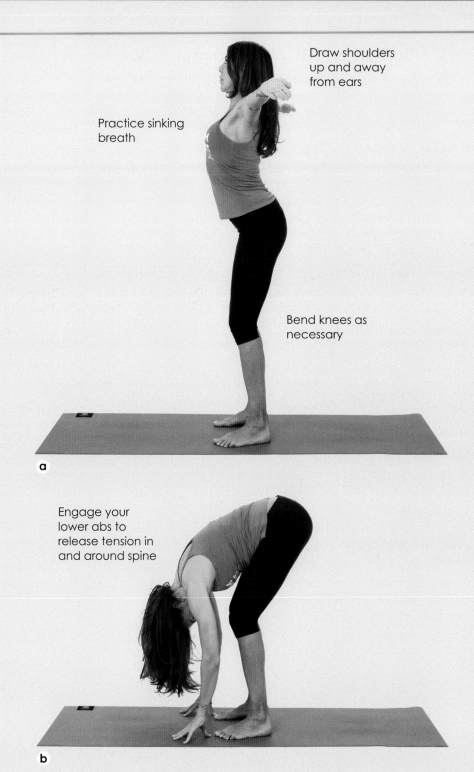

Draw shoulders up and away from ears

Practice sinking breath

Bend knees as necessary

a

Engage your lower abs to release tension in and around spine

b

Use standing forward fold in mountain I as a transition pose. Or, use it in mountain II as a place to hold and breathe, stretching your low back and middle back.

## Getting Into the Pose

Place your feet hip-width apart. Raise your arms overhead, bend your knees, and fold forward, leading with your chest. Extend your arms to the side as you bring your hands to the floor (figure a). The spine stays in neutral until the belly and thighs meet, after which the spine can move into flexion. For a greater challenge, if your low back feels supported, grab your elbows and frame your face.

## Holding the Pose

Keep your knees bent to protect your low back (figure b). Engage your abdominal muscles as you lift your tailbone to the sky. Shake out your head and neck to release tension. Direct your breath into your back or hamstrings, wherever you feel the most tension.

## Modification

If you have tight hamstrings or concerns about your low back, place your hands on a block for support.

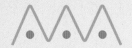

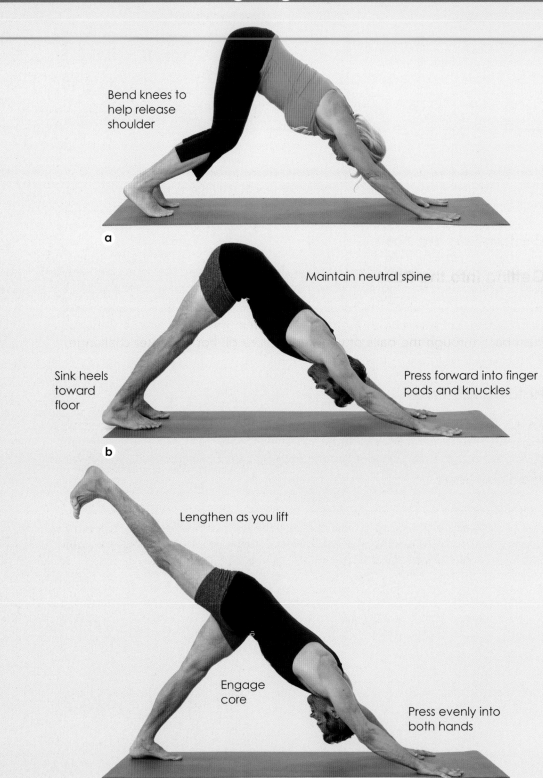

Bend knees to help release shoulder

**a**

Maintain neutral spine

Sink heels toward floor

Press forward into finger pads and knuckles

**b**

Lengthen as you lift

Engage core

Press evenly into both hands

**c**

Downward-facing dog (also called down dog) is the cornerstone of a flow yoga practice, as you saw in the flow series and will see again in the workouts in chapter 10. This pose is an excellent transition between other poses and provides strength and flexibility exactly where you need it. Use this pose often in mountains I, II, and III.

## Getting Into the Pose

From child's pose, reach forward with your hands and press them into the mat with your fingers spread wide (figure a). Lift your hips into an inverted V shape. Push back through the balls of your feet (figure b). For a greater challenge, lift one leg at a time to the sky (figure c).

## Holding the Pose

Keep your head between your arms as you lift your tailbone to the sky. Sink your heels toward the floor without rounding your back.

## Modifications

If your back rounds, bend your knees. Remember that this is a forward fold, and most people will need to bend their knees to some degree in order to keep the back from rounding. If you have shoulder or wrist concerns, remain in an extended child's pose or dolphin pose (described next).

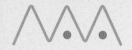

## Dolphin

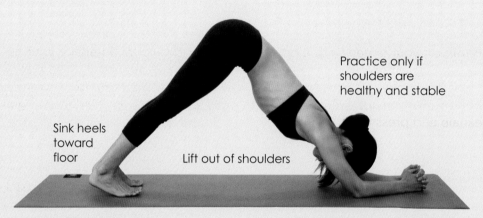

Sink heels toward floor

Lift out of shoulders

Practice only if shoulders are healthy and stable

Press into forearms

It's common to have imbalances in your upper body because you either favor one arm (especially true for athletes) or neglect working your upper body altogether. Dolphin pose is a great way to build strength and flexibility in and around your shoulders. Use this pose in mountains II and III.

## Getting Into the Pose

Begin on your knees, with elbows above your shoulders. Interlace your fingers and press your forearms into the floor. Curl your toes and lift your hips, pushing into the forearms and shifting your body towards the back of the mat. For the swimming dolphin, inhale and draw your face over your hands. Then exhale and press back.

## Holding the Pose

Slowly straighten your legs as you sink your heels toward the floor. Look back at your toes, and press the floor away with your arms. Lift your shoulders away from your ears.

## Modification

If your back rounds, bend your knees.

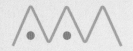

## Airplane

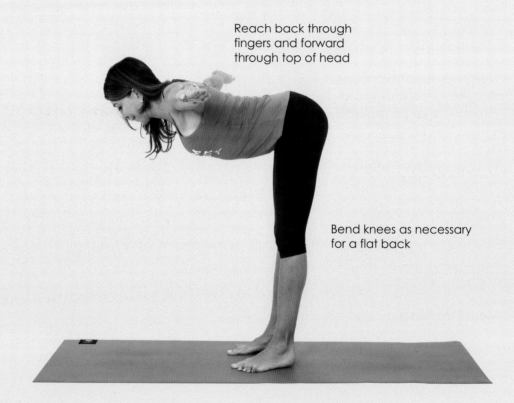

Reach back through
fingers and forward
through top of head

Bend knees as necessary
for a flat back

Airplane pose is ideal to use between forward bends and backbends to elongate and stabilize the spine. Use it during mountains I or II.

## Getting Into the Pose

Standing, raise your arms overhead. Lower your arms to shoulder height, and draw them back. With a slight bend in your knees, hinge forward halfway while maintaining a neutral spine (flat back). Draw your shoulder blades together, and turn your palms toward the floor.

## Holding the Pose

Visualize pulling energy from your chest to your fingertips, keeping your back flat. Look down at the floor, and reach forward through the top of your head. Lift your arms high to move your shoulder blades toward your spine.

## Modifications

If you have low-back concerns, sciatica, or tight hamstrings, bend your knees deeply or place your hands on your thighs.

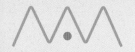

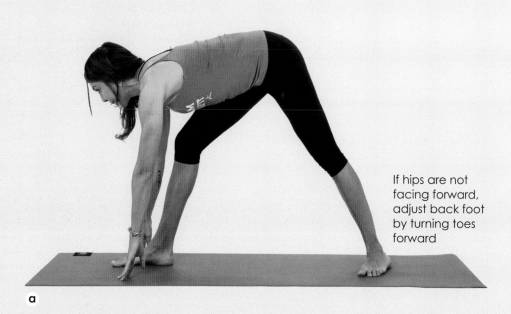

If hips are not facing forward, adjust back foot by turning toes forward

a

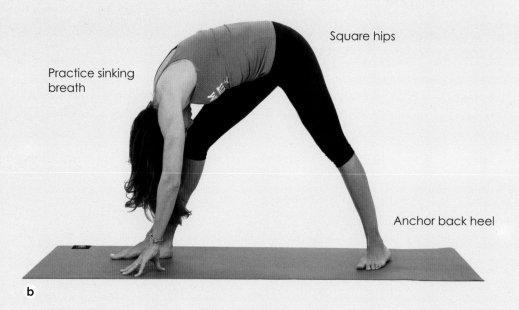

Square hips

Practice sinking breath

Anchor back heel

b

Because your feet are in the same position here as for twisting triangle pose, pyramid pose often precedes or follows that pose in mountain II (figure a). A longer exhalation tells your nervous system it's time to relax. Practice sinking breath (see chapter 3) to help release tightness in your hamstrings.

## Getting Into the Pose

From a short warrior I stance (see chapter 6), square your hips, and hinge forward over your front leg, connecting your belly to the front thigh and elongating the back into the stretch.

## Holding the Pose

Keep your back heel anchored to the mat, and soften your front knee. Focus on the sensation in your hamstrings as you hold the pose and breathe. Tighten your quadriceps for more strength and stability (figure b).

## Modifications

To accommodate tight hamstrings, bend your front knee as necessary or place your hands on a block in front of your front foot.

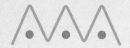

# Standing Chest Expansion With Forward Fold

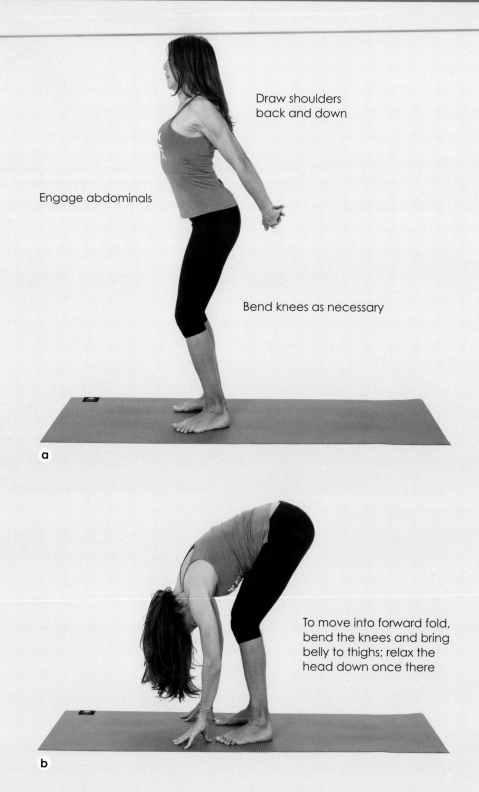

Draw shoulders back and down

Engage abdominals

Bend knees as necessary

a

To move into forward fold, bend the knees and bring belly to thighs; relax the head down once there

b

**STRENGTHENS:**
abdominal muscles • upper back
**STRETCHES:**
hamstrings • chest • shoulders

The chest muscles are some of the tightest muscles in the Western body. Poor posture, indicated by rounded shoulders and a forward head posture, contributes to many problems such as back and neck pain, tension in the jaw, headaches, breathing difficulties, and high blood pressure, and it even affects your mood. Spend a little time each day stretching your chest and breathing into an open heart and lungs. Use this pose before, during, and after any upper-body work to stretch shoulders and chest during mountains I, II, or III.

## Getting Into the Pose

From mountain pose, interlace your fingers behind your back and straighten your arms (figure a). Slowly raise your arms, bend your knees, and lower into a forward fold, leading with your chest.

## Holding the Pose

Breathe into your shoulders. Lift your tailbone to the sky, and tighten your abdominal muscles. Drop your head, but lift your shoulders away from your ears while keeping the wrists stacked over the shoulders (figure b). Let every breath guide you deeper into the stretch.

## Modifications

For low-back concerns, particularly disc injury or sciatica, remain standing with your knees slightly bent. If you're unable to clasp your fingers, use a strap or a hand towel.

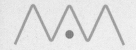

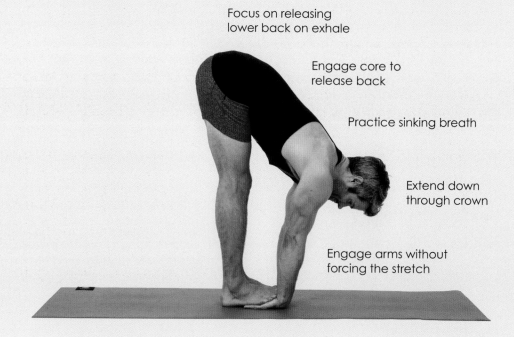

Focus on releasing
lower back on exhale

Engage core to
release back

Practice sinking breath

Extend down
through crown

Engage arms without
forcing the stretch

This pose is effective after sun salutations or following the flow series in mountain II to offset the position of the wrists in plank, crocodile, and upward-facing dog as well as stretch the back side of the body and strengthen the feet.

## Getting Into the Pose

**Gorilla:** From a standing forward fold, wrap your big toes with your index and middle fingers. Bring your elbows out to each side. Inhale and look up, straightening your spine while pressing your feet and toes into the ground. Exhaling, draw the top of your head toward your feet.

**Wrist stretch:** From gorilla pose flip your hands so that your palms face up. Slide your hands beneath your feet until your toes meet the insides of your wrists. Gently shift your weight forward toward your toes. Inhale and look up, straightening your spine. Exhaling, draw the top of your head toward your feet.

## Holding the Pose

In both gorilla pose and the wrist stretch, slowly straighten your legs until you find a comfortable stretch.

## Modifications

For low-back concerns, particularly disc injury or sciatica, place your hands on your thighs. Also place your hands on your thighs if you're unable to reach the floor. Remember to always bend your knees in forward folds.

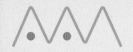

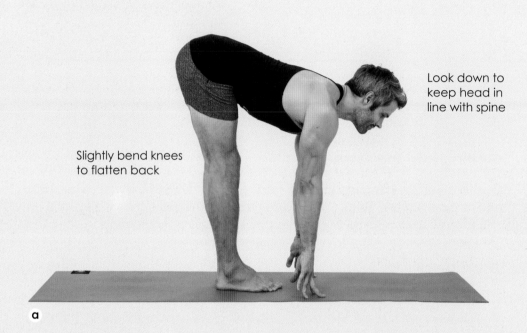

Look down to keep head in line with spine

Slightly bend knees to flatten back

a

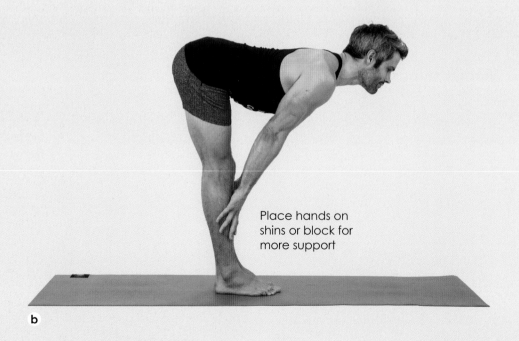

Place hands on shins or block for more support

b

Monkey pose is effective in mountain I or II as a complement to forward bends. This pose activates the back, improving your posture and core strength.

## Getting Into the Pose

From a standing forward fold, place your fingertips on the floor in front of your feet. Inhaling, lift your chest away from your thighs, pulling the shoulder blades together, bending the knees as needed to maintain a straight spine (figure a). Hold, or exhale back to the forward fold.

## Holding the Pose

Look slightly forward, keeping your back flat.

## Modifications

For low-back concerns, particularly disc injury or sciatica, place your hands on your thighs. If you can't flatten your back with your fingertips on the floor, place your hands on your shins with your knees bent (figure b).

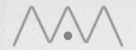

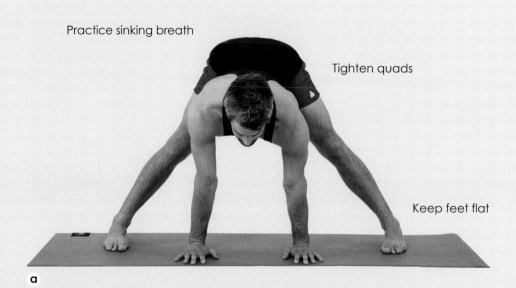

Practice sinking breath

Tighten quads

Keep feet flat

a

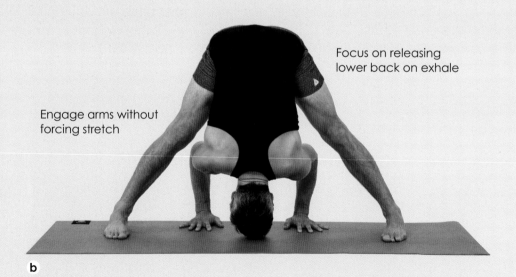

Focus on releasing lower back on exhale

Engage arms without forcing stretch

b

Use this pose in mountain II when your hamstrings are warm enough for a deep stretch.

## Getting Into the Pose

Stand with your feet apart and toes facing forward. Place your palms flat on the floor (bending the knees as needed). Push your feet out, keeping the soles flat on the mat (figure *a*). For an added challenge, grab your big toes with your index and middle fingers, or interlace your fingers above your head for a chest expansion.

## Holding the Pose

Firm your quadriceps while extending the crown of your head toward the floor (figure *b*).

## Modification

If you have an ankle or groin injury, use caution with this pose and listen to your body, choosing positions that honor where you are in your recovery.

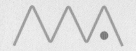

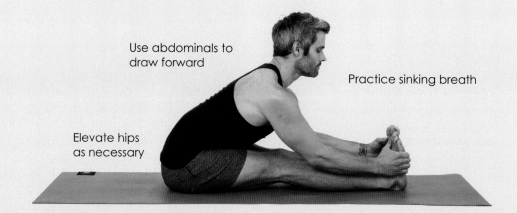

Use abdominals to
draw forward

Practice sinking breath

Elevate hips
as necessary

This pose is used often in fitness as the benchmark for flexibility. As such, some people tend to become competitive, grab their feet, and pull themselves forward. This forceful action causes great harm to the low back and does nothing to lengthen the muscles. Remember the YogaFit essence of *listening to your body; and letting go of expectations, judgments, and your competitive spirit.* Draw forward from a desire to let go, not to win a competition. Use this pose in mountain III when your body is thoroughly warm.

## Getting Into the Pose

From a seated position, extend your legs. Pull your toes back toward your body. Reach forward, placing your hands on your legs, ankles, or feet, or on the floor. Draw forward through the top of your head, lengthening your low back and connecting the belly to the thighs. For an added challenge, bend one knee, bringing your foot flat to the floor with the toes pointing forward. Keeping your knee pointing straight up, reach forward.

## Holding the Pose

Using a sinking breath (see chapter 3), continue to reach forward toward your feet with your chest and the crown of your head. Firm your quadriceps. Relax your shoulders back and down, and enjoy the stretch.

## Modifications

If you have tight hamstrings, sit on a folded blanket or rolled-up yoga mat, use a strap or hand towel around your feet, or bend your knees. For a more restorative option, use a rolled-up mat, blanket, or egg blocks under the thighs to support your bent knees. Release forward, and breathe deeply. Supporting the body can allow for more relaxation.

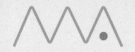

Practice sinking breath

Point toes
straight up

Elevate hips
as necessary

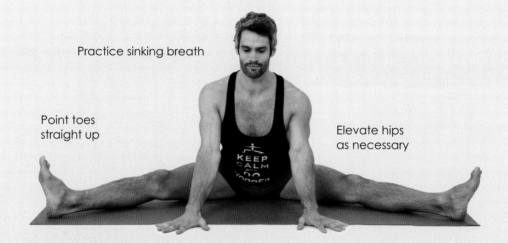

Use seated straddle splits during mountain III after your body is thoroughly warm.

## Getting Into the Pose

From a seated position, spread your legs wide. Hinge at your hips, place your hands on the floor in front of you, and use your abdominal muscles to draw forward while keeping your back straight as possible until you have hinged as far forward as possible.

## Holding the Pose

Breathe into your back. Pull your toes back toward your body, and point them toward the sky. Bend your knees as necessary. Relax into the fold by releasing the head down.

## Modifications

If you have tight hamstrings, sit on a folded blanket or rolled-up yoga mat, or bend your knees.

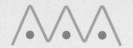

## Cat and Cow

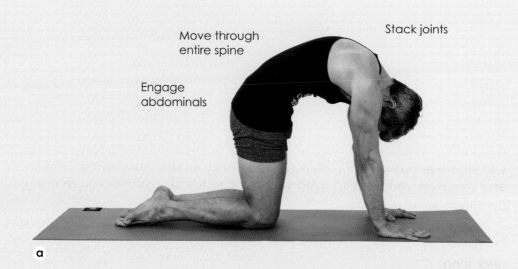

Move through
entire spine

Stack joints

Engage
abdominals

a

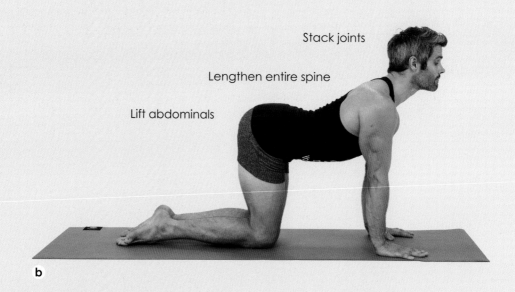

Stack joints

Lengthen entire spine

Lift abdominals

b

Flow the cat and cow poses with your breathing to warm up your torso and spine in mountain I. Or, hold each pose individually in mountain II or III.

## Getting Into the Pose

**Cat (figure a):** From your hands and knees, with your shoulders over your wrists and hips over your knees, round your back to the sky, focusing on drawing the navel to the spine.

**Cow (figure b):** From cat pose, arch your back, reaching the center of the chest forward, and lift through the crown of the head to keep the back of the neck long.

## Holding the Pose

Keep your abdominal muscles firm. In mountain II, focus on lengthening through your entire spine, not just rounding (cat) or arching (cow) your low back.

## Modifications

If you have wrist discomfort or injuries, use fists for wrists with the palms facing each other. For sensitive knees or other knee concerns, use a kneepad for comfort.

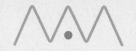

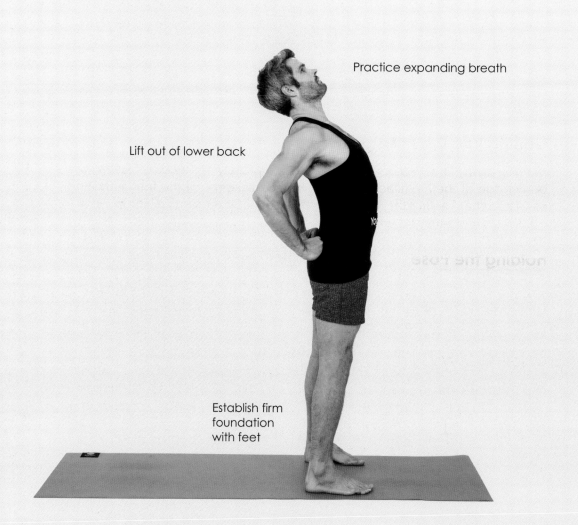

Practice expanding breath

Lift out of lower back

Establish firm
foundation
with feet

**STRENGTHENS:**
  gluteal muscles • lower back
**STRETCHES:**
  chest • shoulders • hip flexors •
  abdominal muscles

Improve flexibility in your spine by extending into a standing backbend. You'll feel the benefits immediately. Perform this pose near the end of mountain II so that your body is very warm.

## Getting Into the Pose

Moving slowly, firm your gluteal muscles and place your hands or fists on the bony ridge of the hip (iliac bone). Begin the backbend at the feet activating pada bandha. Feeling the strength of the legs, lift the chest while firmly dropping the shoulders back and down.

## Holding the Pose

Lift out of your low back, drawing your elbows back to expand your chest. Look toward the sky without dropping your head back. Use expanding breath (see chapter 3) to deepen the sensation.

## Modifications

If you have a low-back injury, do this pose with caution or use the standing chest expansion with forward fold as an alternative. If your neck fatigues, look forward, tucking your chin slightly.

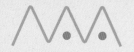

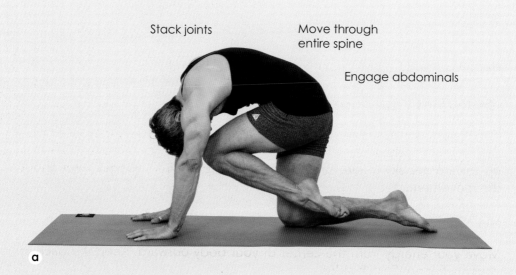

Stack joints

Move through entire spine

Engage abdominals

a

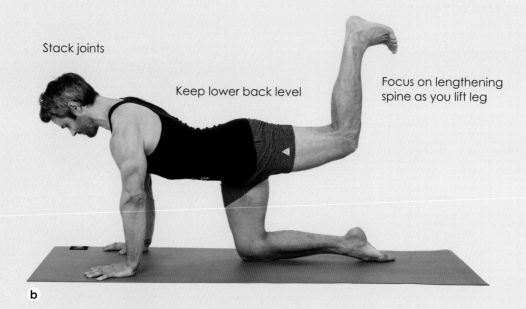

Stack joints

Keep lower back level

Focus on lengthening spine as you lift leg

b

Do sunbird pose in mountain II or III to build strength.

## Getting Into the Pose

From your hands and knees, exhale as you bring one knee under your body toward your forehead (figure *a*). Then inhaling, extend the same leg back and up toward the sky (figure *b*). Contract your abdominal muscles throughout the movement.

## Holding the Pose

Move your energy from the center of your body outward. Keep the back of your neck long. Switch sides.

## Modifications

If you have wrist discomfort or injuries, use fists for wrists with palms facing each other. For sensitive knees or other knee concerns, use kneepads for comfort.

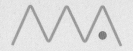

## Camel

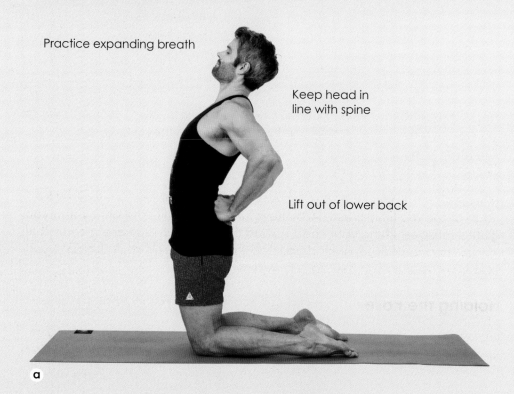

Practice expanding breath

Keep head in
line with spine

Lift out of lower back

a

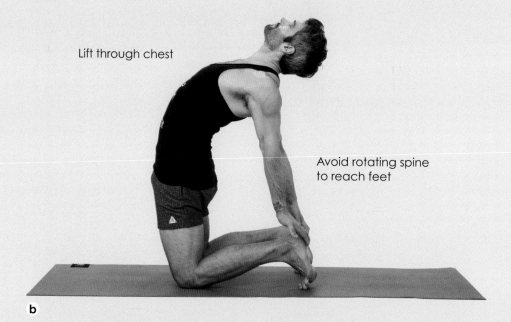

Lift through chest

Avoid rotating spine
to reach feet

b

Similar to standing backbend, this pose works best when your body is warm. Because you're on your knees, use this pose in mountain III.

## Getting Into the Pose

Moving slowly from a kneeling position, place your hands or fists on the bony ridge of the hip (iliac crest). Activate your inner thighs, and gently firm your gluteal muscles, lifting your chest toward the sky (figure *a*). For a greater challenge, drop your arms behind you and grab your heels while keeping your bottom rib in line with the hips and knees (figure *b*).

## Holding the Pose

Lift out of your low back, drawing your elbows back to expand your chest. Look toward the sky without dropping your head back. Use expanding breath in this pose to deepen the sensation.

## Modifications

If you have a low-back injury, use caution with this pose or else, from a kneeling position, interlace your hands behind your back to stretch your chest in the modified version of standing chest expansion with forward fold. If your neck fatigues or you feel dizzy, look forward and tuck your chin slightly. For sensitive knees or other knee concerns, use a kneepad for comfort.

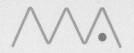

## Locust and Superman

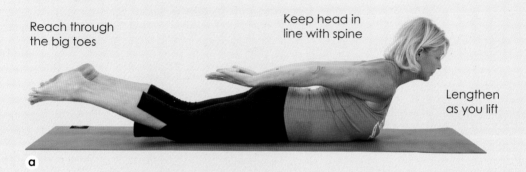

Reach through the big toes

Keep head in line with spine

Lengthen as you lift

a

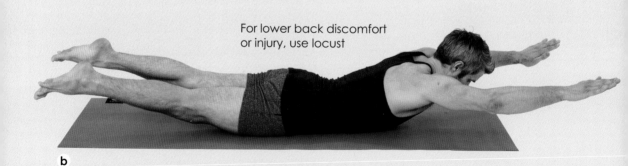

For lower back discomfort or injury, use locust

b

Locust pose works well in mountain III to safely stabilize and strengthen your low back; it's a great pose to ward off back pain and injuries. Superman pose offers the same benefits as locust when done in mountain III but it places more load on the low back, so practice this pose only when your back is healthy and stable. Experiment with Superman pose, picking the modification that builds strength without strain.

## Getting Into the Pose

**Locust (figure *a*):** Lie on your belly with your arms at your sides, palms up. Engage your abdominal muscles and gluteal muscles as you lift your upper and lower body off the ground.

**Superman (figure *b*):** Lie on your belly with your arms stretched above your head. Reach forward, engaging your abdominal muscles and gluteal muscles as you lift your upper and lower body off the ground.

## Holding the Pose

In locust pose and Superman pose, focus on lengthening more than lifting. Become longer with each breath. In locust pose, reach forward through the crown of your head and back through your toes; in the Superman, reach forward with your fingers and back through your toes.

## Modifications

If you're a beginner or if you have a low-back injury, start these poses by folding your arms in front of your face and resting your forehead on your forearms in front of you. From this position, lift one leg at a time. Or lift just your upper body or just your lower body. As you develop strength and can hold these modifications for 5 to 10 breaths, try locust and then Superman.

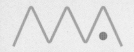

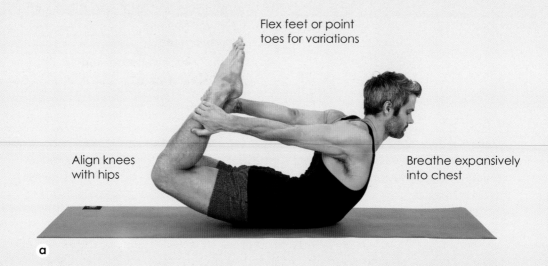

Flex feet or point
toes for variations

Align knees
with hips

Breathe expansively
into chest

**a**

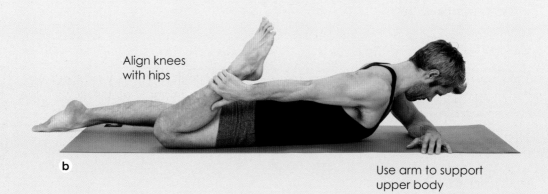

Align knees
with hips

**b**

Use arm to support
upper body

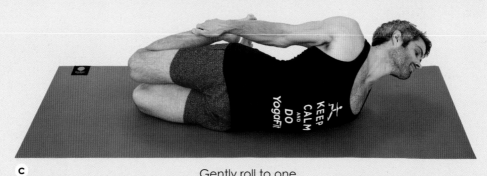

Press ankles against hands

**c**

Gently roll to one
side on exhalation

Bow pose and half bow pose create tension in order to release pent-up energy. Notice how relaxed and invigorated you feel after the effort of holding these poses for 5 to 10 breaths in mountain III.

## Getting Into the Pose

**Bow (figure *a*):** Lying on your belly, grab your right ankle with your right hand and your left ankle with your left hand. Lift your chest and legs to the sky. Pull your ankles back against your hands with your feet flexed or pointed, as if straightening your legs.

**Half bow (figure *b*):** Hold one ankle at a time, flexing or pointing your foot. Switch sides.

**Side bow (figure *c*):** From bow pose, maintain the dynamic tension by pressing the ankles against the hands and activating the inner thighs to keep the ankle, knees, and hips in line. Breathing into the chest and shoulders, gently roll to one side on the exhalation. Hold for 5 to 10 breaths, then on the inhalation, roll back through bow and switch sides.

## Holding the Pose

Keep breathing into your chest as you open more with each inhalation and lengthen out of your low back.

## Modification

If you can't reach your ankles, use straps around your ankles. For a more restorative option in half bow, rest your forehead on the forearm and focus on lifting the knee away from the floor gently.

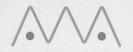

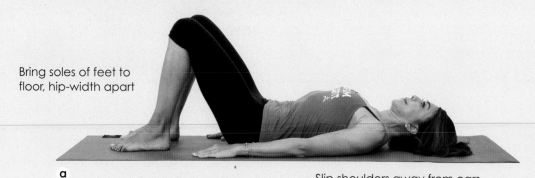

Bring soles of feet to floor, hip-width apart

Slip shoulders away from ears

a

Stack knees over ankles

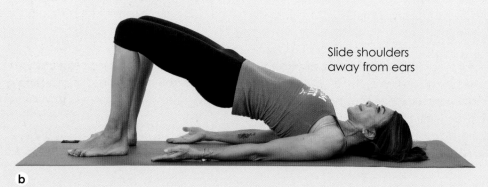

Slide shoulders away from ears

b

Engage inner thighs to keep knees stacked over ankles

Focus on a deep, expansive breath

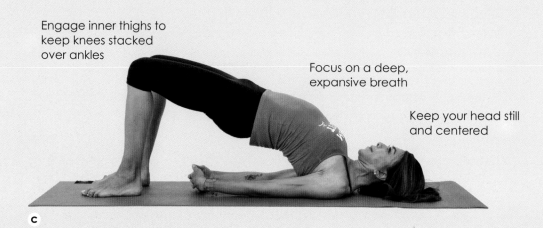

Keep your head still and centered

c

**STRENGTHENS:**
gluteal muscles • hamstrings • hip adductors • lower back

**STRETCHES:**
hip flexors • abdominal muscles • chest • shoulders

Bridge pose is an excellent way to stretch the front of your hips and open your chest, particularly if you sit for long periods or regularly walk, run, or cycle. This pose also targets muscles deep in your low back and hips that are difficult to reach when upright. Move up and down with your breathing in mountain I, or hold in mountain III.

## Getting Into the Pose

Lie on your back with your palms down. Slide your shoulders away from your ears. Bring the soles of your feet to the floor, hip-width apart (figure *a*). Press through your feet to lift your hips (figure *b*). For a greater challenge, interlace your fingers under your body. Walk your shoulders toward each other so that your body is resting on the outside edges of your shoulders. Look toward your chest or the sky while focusing on your breath (figure *c*). For more challenge, shift your weight into the right foot while lifting the left foot into the air and hold for five breaths. Switch sides.

## Holding the Pose

Keep your head still to protect your neck (i.e., don't look around). Use your inner thighs to keep your knees in line with your hips and toes. Breathe deeply into your open chest and navel.

## Modification

Turn your palms up for more chest opening and core focus (figure *b*).

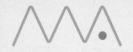

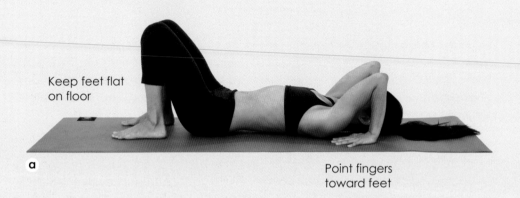

Keep feet flat
on floor

**a**

Point fingers
toward feet

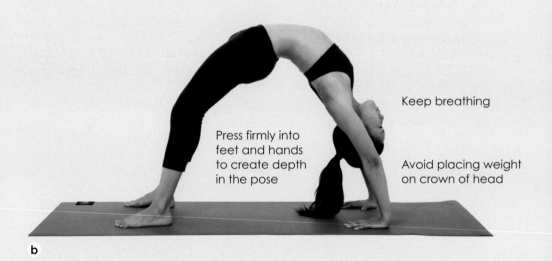

Keep breathing

Press firmly into
feet and hands
to create depth
in the pose

Avoid placing weight
on crown of head

**b**

**STRENGTHENS:**
gluteal muscles • hamstrings • lower back • upper back • shoulders

**STRETCHES:**
hip flexors • abdominal muscles • chest • shoulders

Although you're in a backbend position, wheel pose is more of a shoulder opener than a backbend. Practice downward-facing dog, dolphin, or bridge in order to prepare for this energizing pose. Do this pose near the end of mountain III when your body and mind are primed for a big stretch and a natural pick-me-up.

## Getting Into the Pose

After bridge pose or from bridge pose, place both your hands on either side of your ears and point your fingers toward your feet. Place your feet flat on the floor hip-width apart (figure a). Press through your hands to lift your head and shoulders off the floor. Straighten your arms first, then your legs (figure b).

## Holding the Pose

Focus on stretching the front of your body without struggle or strain. To come out of the backbend, tuck your chin to your chest and slowly place the back of your head on the mat as you return to the starting position. Bring your knees to your chest, and relax.

## Modifications

To build strength for wheel pose, keep your elbows bent and only come to the top of your head. Keep all your weight on your hands and feet (*not* your head and neck). Practice several push-ups, each one higher than the last. Come down slowly on the back of your head as you lower your back to your mat. Bring your knees to your chest, and relax.

# CHAPTER

# Twists

A healthy spine moves in all directions, and your spinal work in YogaFit is not complete without twisting. Twists have a reputation for delivering instant gratification; their effects are felt almost immediately. Done properly and after the body is warm, twisting poses target highly specialized muscles in the torso, building strength while releasing tension from deep within your body.

Twisting poses likely affect more than just your spine. Twists can be detoxifying. Yogis claim that through rotation and the resulting compression of the internal organs you stimulate the organs of your abdomen and pelvis by wringing out old blood and excess fluid, allowing fresh blood and oxygen to flow in on release. Further, compressing and manipulating your intestines through twisting poses also improves digestion and elimination. The best way to know if these claims are true is to try them and listen to your body, noticing the changes that occur through your practice.

Twisting is also very energizing and wonderful for creating heat in yoga practice, allowing for greater release of tension. Consider a flowing twist in mountain II (e.g., a kneeling lunge twist or twisting chair), before deeper, more releasing twists in mountain III. Use a one-breath, one-movement pattern and flow gently from side to side 3 to 4 times before holding the twist for 3 to 5 breaths each side. Allow the range of motion of the twist to very gently become greater.

There are different schools of thought when it comes to twists and where they start. You may hear some teachers cueing to allow the hips to come along in the twist to keep pressure out of the lower back, while others will insist that the hips stay squared to allow for more a pure rotation in the spine. Both ways can be safe when done properly without force, but the results will differ. When the hips are allowed to move (compensation), the student can twist further to the side without pressure in the hips and back, but that is because of the compensation. When the hips are kept anchored, there may appear to be less range of motion and the movement is kept in the torso. If your goal is to increase your true range of motion, then keeping the hips squared and moving without force is a good choice. However, if keeping the hips squared and twisting causes discomfort, then allowing some give in the hips would be appropriate.

Proper alignment is critical to keeping the spine safe in twisting postures. Before moving into any twisting pose, create space in your spine by practicing some of the YogaFit's seven principles of alignment (SPA) from chapter 2. Doing so should ensure the safest possible position for smooth and healthy movement. The SPA that pertain to twists are as follows:

- **Establish a base and dynamic tension (SPA 1).** The lumbar spine does not twist very much, so it is helpful to think of twists beginning just above the navel and, like the stripe on a barbershop pole, twists wind up to the cervical spine.

  This upward spiral needs to be supported by a strong base and the bandhas. By anchoring your feet while drawing energy up through the arches of your feet (pada bandha) and into the pelvic floor (mula bandha) in standing poses such as twisting triangle, and by keeping the base of your pelvis (sit bones; ischial tuberosities) anchored in seated twists, you support your pelvis. Through establishing a reliable foundation, rotation remains where you need it—in your spine.

  Remember that a strong base is not the same as a rigid base. Keeping the breath full and smooth while bandhas are softly engaged will set the stage for a delicious twist.

- **Create core stability (SPA 2).** Before moving into any rotation, engage the bandhas. Along with mula bandha and pada bandha mentioned earlier, uddiyana bandha (the contraction of the transverse abdominals) further supports the spine in twists. All twists should be initiated from a strong core, allowing the oblique abdominal muscles and other torso muscles to drive the action instead. Avoid using your arms as leverage too soon.

- **Align the spine (SPA 3).** Before moving into any rotation, your spine must be in neutral position. This position allows the vertebrae to rotate safely and smoothly on top of one another without pinching nerves or injuring the discs. You will notice that as your deep core muscles (bandhas) are activated the spine will lengthen and elevate, creating the alignment needed to twist safely.

- **Relax the shoulders back and down (SPA 5).** Drawing your shoulder blades down and back helps align your spine and engage your core.

Always exercise attention and caution when practicing any form of rotation. Attend particularly to the position of your head and neck. It is common when rotating your head to also tilt it forward, backward, or to one side. Tilting can aggravate your neck, leading to tension or even injury. So, when twisting, you might try using mirrors to ensure that your head remains in line with your spine (SPA 3). Of course, if turning your head one direction is uncomfortable in a pose, look straight ahead or even in the opposite direction. As long as you're in alignment and out of pain, your body will benefit.

In addition to the SPA, a couple other principles come into play when practicing twists.

• **Lead with your gut (belly) as opposed to your head (neck).** As mentioned, all twists begin with the contraction of the oblique abdominal muscles in the waist and slowly move upward. The temptation in rotation is to set your sights on a deeper twist by turning your head first. However, because your neck is more flexible than the rest of your spine, your torso can't follow, and you're stuck with frustration. Rather than releasing tension, twisting in this way creates more tension. To make matters worse, you sometimes use an arm to pull yourself deeper into a twisting pose rather than relaxing and allowing rotation to occur when your body is ready.

• **Relax, and let your breath be your guide.** With each inhalation, continue to lengthen your backbone; with each exhalation, soften into the spaciousness twisting allows. When you let go of forcing things and focus on the process rather than on a final prize or goal, you gain much more.

All twists should be performed only when the body is thoroughly warm—in other words, within mountains II or III.

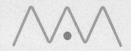

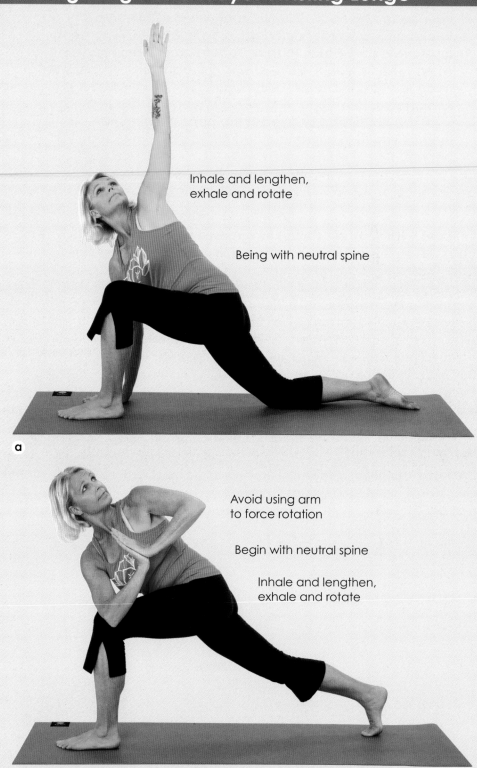

Inhale and lengthen, exhale and rotate

Being with neutral spine

a

Avoid using arm to force rotation

Begin with neutral spine

Inhale and lengthen, exhale and rotate

b

Practice twisting lunge and prayer twisting lunge during mountain II when your body is thoroughly warm.

## Getting Into the Pose

**Twisting lunge (figure *a*):** From a lunge position with your left foot forward, place your right hand on the floor close to your left foot. With a straight spine, sweep your left arm up, reaching toward the sky.

**Prayer twisting lunge (figure *b*):** From a kneeling lunge, place your hands in prayer position over your chest. Rotate, placing the back of your arm against the outside of your forward thigh. Lift your back knee off the mat, and look upward. Keep the top shoulder back and down.

## Holding the Pose

Press through your back heel, and stack your forward knee over your ankle. Keep your chest close to your front knee as you twist from the waist. Look up. Switch sides.

## Modifications

For less intensity, drop your back knee to the mat in a kneeling lunge. Place your bottom hand on a block to lift your chest, and bring your spine into neutral position for rotation.

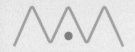

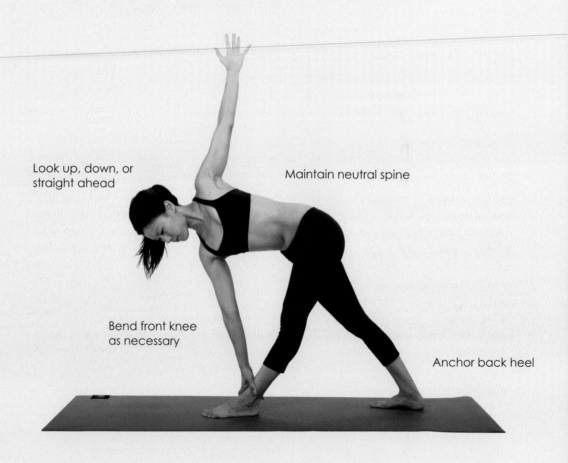

Look up, down, or straight ahead

Maintain neutral spine

Bend front knee as necessary

Anchor back heel

Twisting triangle pose is a challenging pose that combines elements of forward folding, balancing, and twisting. Because the foot position is the same, twisting triangle typically follows pyramid pose in mountain II.

## Getting Into the Pose

From a short warrior I stance, turn your back toes in until they nearly face the front of your mat. Square your hips, and hinge forward over your front leg, keeping a microbend in your front knee. If your left foot is in front, reach your right hand toward the left knee and slide toward the floor, keeping the spine straight. Twist to the left, placing your left hand on the left hip and then, for more sensation, reaching your left arm to the sky.

## Holding the Pose

Keep your back heel anchored to the mat as you slowly straighten your legs. Lengthen your spine (rather than round forward) as you open your chest to the sky. Look up to your left hand or down or straight ahead. Switch sides.

## Modifications

Bend your front knee or place your hand on a block to accommodate tight hamstrings. If you have a disc injury, use extra caution in this pose; the injury could be aggravated. Use pyramid pose as an alternative if necessary.

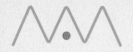

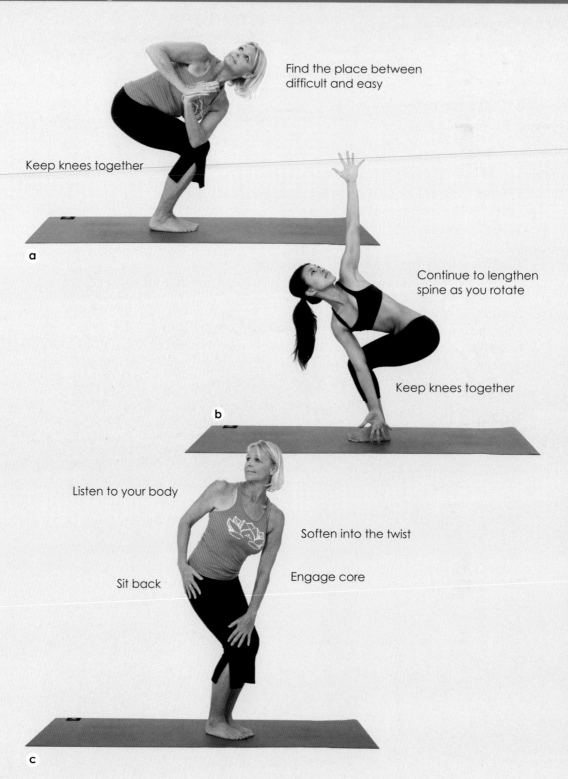

Find the place between difficult and easy

Keep knees together

a

Continue to lengthen spine as you rotate

Keep knees together

b

Listen to your body

Soften into the twist

Sit back

Engage core

c

Practice this variation of chair pose only in mountain II; it requires extra attention to alignment to prevent injuring your low back.

## Getting Into the Pose

Start chair pose with your feet and knees together. Lengthen your spine, and place your hands over your chest in prayer position. Twist from the waist, placing your elbow on the outside of your opposite thigh (figure *a*). For an added challenge, touch your bottom hand to the floor outside your foot. Reach up with your top arm as you roll your chest toward the sky (figure *b*).

When you're first learning this pose, begin with a modified version in which you place one hand on your opposite thigh and the other on your lower back or hip, focusing on keeping your knees together and your hips back (figure *c*).

## Holding the Pose

Engage your core to support your low back. Inhale to lengthen; exhale to twist. Keep your knees together as you release deeper into rotation.

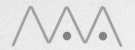

## Side Crow

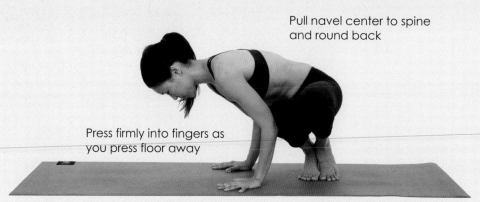

Pull navel center to spine and round back

Press firmly into fingers as you press floor away

**a**

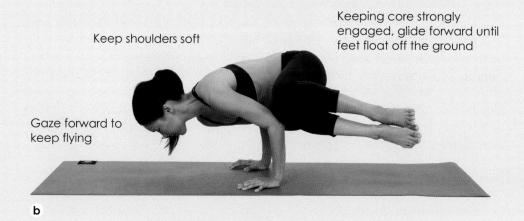

Keep shoulders soft

Keeping core strongly engaged, glide forward until feet float off the ground

Gaze forward to keep flying

**b**

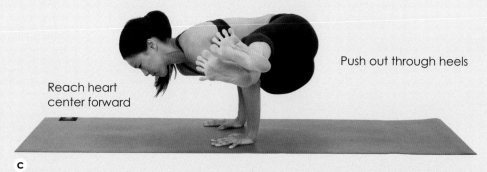

Breathe strongly into back

Push out through heels

Reach heart center forward

**c**

**STRENGTHENS:**
chest • arms • shoulders •
obliques • core
**STRETCHES:**
back • oblique abdominal
muscles • gluteal muscles

Once you have practiced twisting chair and feel as if you have enough space in twisting chair, side crow in mountain phases II or III will give added challenge and increase the twisting sensation while at the same time strengthening the core and upper body.

## Getting Into the Pose

From twisting chair toward the right, lift the heels and drop the tailbone lower. Place the left triceps on the outside of the right thigh with the hands moving from prayer position to the floor shoulder-width apart. Press through the fingers to activate hasta bandha (figure *a*). Pressing the legs together, pull the abdominal muscles strongly toward the spine as you shift weight onto your hands. Continue to glide forward until the feet gently lift off the floor (figure *b*). For more sensation, slowly straighten the legs and push through the heels, keeping the gaze forward (figure *c*).

## Holding the Pose

Continue pressing the floor away from you, and breathe into your broadening back. Keep the breath slow, deep, and steady.

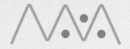

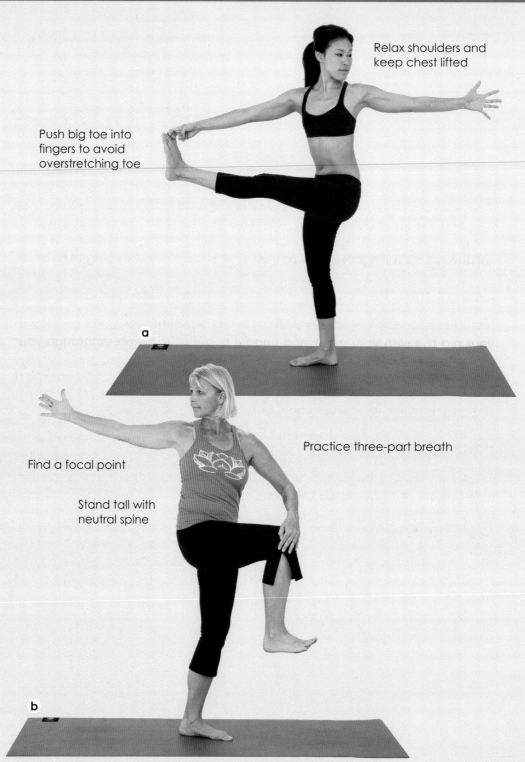

Relax shoulders and keep chest lifted

Push big toe into fingers to avoid overstretching toe

**a**

Practice three-part breath

Find a focal point

Stand tall with neutral spine

**b**

With the added element of rotation in a standing balance pose, you get twice the challenge and twice the benefit. Use this two-for-one pose in valley II. Keep in mind that trying harder only makes the pose more difficult. Trade in willpower for a willingness to relax; trust in your body's innate ability to balance.

## Getting Into the Pose

Standing tall in a mountain pose, lift your left leg. With your right hand, grasp your big toe with your index and middle fingers. Slowly press through your heel to straighten your leg, and twist to the left (figure a). In order to keep the spine safe in this twisting posture, you should be able to bring the knee higher to grasp the toe rather than flex the spine to reach the toe. Work at being able to bring the knee as high as possible before practicing the binding version.

## Holding the Pose

Place your right hand on your hip or open the arm behind you, following with your head. Keep your lower body strong, and focus on your breath.

## Modifications

As pictured in figure b, keep your knee bent (or use a strap) if you're unable to straighten your leg. Use a wall or chair behind you for more support, if necessary.

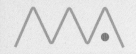

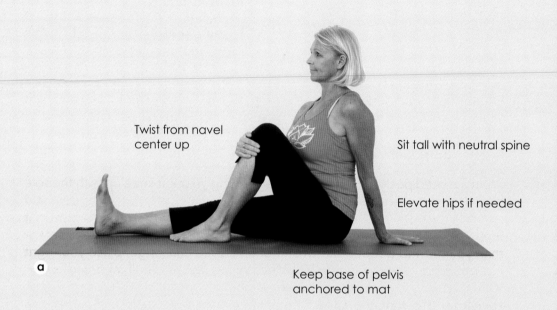

Twist from navel center up

Sit tall with neutral spine

Elevate hips if needed

a

Keep base of pelvis anchored to mat

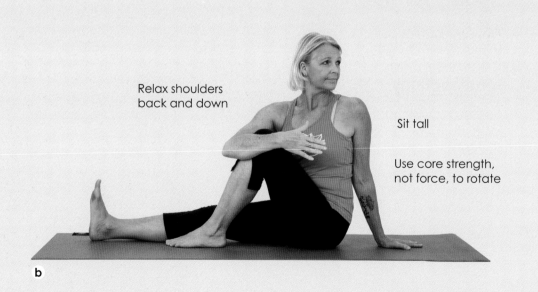

Relax shoulders back and down

Sit tall

Use core strength, not force, to rotate

b

Do this pose in mountain III to release your low back while building strength in and around your spine.

## Getting Into the Pose

From a seated position, extend your legs. Bring your left knee up with the sole of your foot on the floor. Place your left hand next to you or behind you, and sit tall (figure a). Beginning at the navel, rotate to the left, bringing your right forearm around to hold your left shin (figure b). Use your core strength rather than your arm to deepen the twist. For an added challenge, place your right elbow outside your left knee. Hold the position while breathing mindfully.

## Holding the Pose

Use only your core strength to deepen the twist. Lengthen your spine with each inhalation; twist further with each exhalation. Switch sides.

## Modification

If you have difficulty keeping your back straight, sit on a rolled-up yoga mat or folded blanket. Elevating your hips relieves tension caused by tight hamstrings that can tip the pelvis back, making it difficult to sit with a neutral spine.

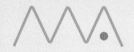

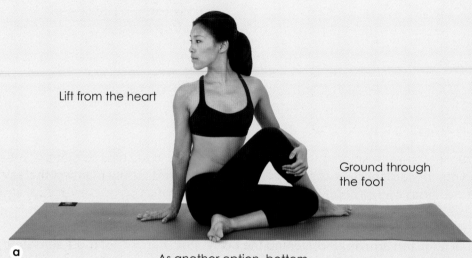

Lift from the heart

Ground through the foot

As another option, bottom leg can remain straight

a

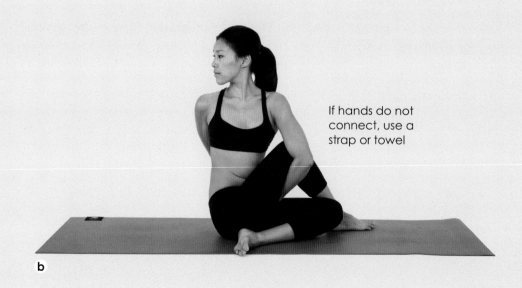

If hands do not connect, use a strap or towel

b

This mountain III pose builds on the previous twist for more rotation and also added stretch in the upper body.

## Getting Into the Pose

From a seated position, bring the left heel in toward the hips so that the knee points forward, and cross the right leg over the left, firmly planting the sole of the right foot on the mat. On an inhalation, sweep the arms upward and lengthen the spine. On the exhalation, turn toward the right, and let the arms relax downward while allowing the left hand to rest on the right shin (figure a). Reach the left arm around, behind the body. Hold here or, for more sensation, reach the left arm through the legs between the outside of the right shin and behind the right thigh, and reach the right hand around the left hip with the hands moving toward one another and clasping (figure b).

## Holding the Pose

Keep the spine reaching upward, and take steady, slow, deep breaths, gently pulling the hands in opposite directions without letting go. Hold for three or four breaths. Follow by releasing the pull and relaxing into the deep stretch.

## Modifications

If the hands don't reach each other and connect, use a strap. If the hips are tight, elevate the pelvis on a rolled-up mat or folded blanket.

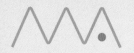

## Turkish Twist

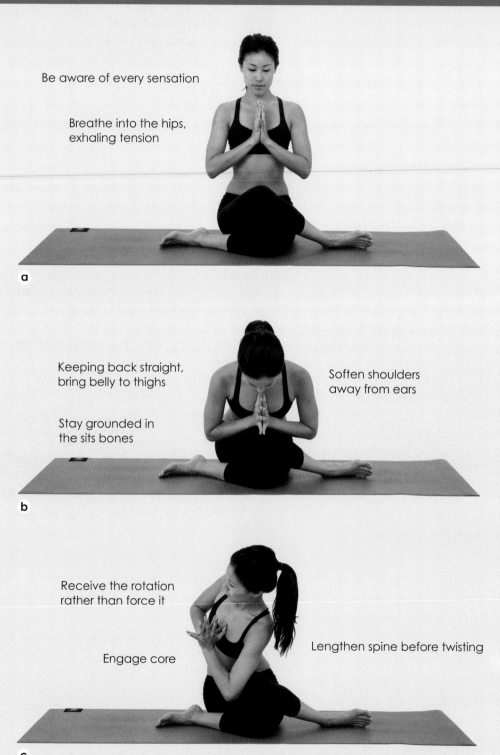

Be aware of every sensation

Breathe into the hips, exhaling tension

**a**

Keeping back straight, bring belly to thighs

Stay grounded in the sits bones

Soften shoulders away from ears

**b**

Receive the rotation rather than force it

Engage core

Lengthen spine before twisting

**c**

This mountain III pose offers all the benefits of rotation combined with a deep hip stretch.

## Getting Into the Pose

Cross one knee over the other. Draw your feet back toward your hips. First, sit tall (figure *a*) and relax into the hip stretch by drawing your forehead toward your knee on the exhalation (figure *b*). Use the sinking breath technique (chapter 3) to help release tension. Then sit tall, and place your hands over your chest in prayer position. Rotate toward your top leg, placing your elbow on your thigh (figure *c*).

## Holding the Pose

Inhale to lengthen; exhale to rotate. Hold for 5 to 10 breaths. Switch sides.

## Modifications

If one hip lifts off the floor, sit on a rolled-up yoga mat or folded blanket. If you have knee pain or difficultly stacking your knees, do a seated spinal twist instead.

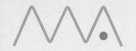

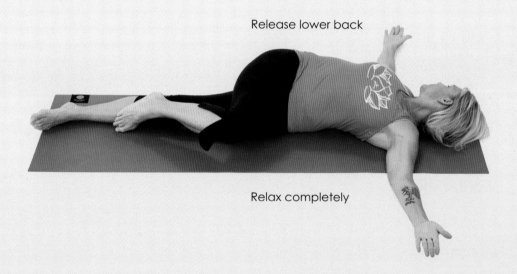

Release lower back

Relax completely

Use this pose to release your low back after standing postures. The pose works well near the end of mountain III to prepare your body for final relaxation pose.

## Getting Into the Pose

Lie down on the floor. From knees to chest pose (see chapter 9), extend your left leg along the floor. Place your right foot on the floor and push to lift, and shift your hips slightly to the right. If needed, use your left hand to gently draw your right knee toward the floor.

## Holding the Pose

Keeping both shoulders on the floor, look to the right. Practice sinking breath for optimal release and relaxation. Switch sides.

## Modifications

If you have a disc injury, the rotation and flexion in this pose might aggravate the injury. In this case, place both feet on the floor and lower your legs together to one side.

# Deep, Relaxing Stretches and Inversions

At the end of a YogaFit workout, as with any physical exercise, your body is warm and your muscles are fatigued. This is the optimal time to practice deep, relaxing stretches and inversions. When you turn up your internal thermostat in mountains I and II, your muscles and connective tissue become more pliable and can lengthen effectively without injury. When you're wrung out both physically and mentally, your mind and body are more willing to relax and release muscular tension caused by strength training (mountain II) or stress. The gentle movement and breath work of a flowing practice can help discharge energy, getting you ready to truly let go of mental and physical stress.

## Deep, Relaxing Stretches

Deep, relaxing stretches are best done in mountain III, the cool-down segment of your YogaFit workout. This chapter includes these stretches:

Child's pose
Kneeling lunge and crescent lunge
Quadriceps stretch
Forward splits
Kneeling shoulder stretch
Revolving knee to head
Sage pose
Frog
Butterfly
Turtle

Upside-down pigeon
Supine half lotus
Knees to chest
Dead bug
Big toe hold
Fish
Final relaxation

These stretching poses are designed to increase flexibility in your muscles and joints and to release stress and tension. Note that the seated forward fold and seated straddle splits from chapter 7 are also considered deep, relaxing stretches and should be incorporated into mountain III.

Two of the primary benefits of deep, relaxing stretches are to maintain functional flexibility and release stress.

• **Maintaining functional flexibility.** Yoga poses are known for requiring exceptional flexibility, but as far as your health is concerned it's far more important to maintain functional flexibility—the ability for your body to move easily through a normal range of motion. Your body's level of functional flexibility is compromised by everything from sports training to the natural aging process. Without regular movement and stretching, your muscles experience atrophy (shrink), and the fascia become sticky and thick, resulting in limited range of motion. More important is that you lose your ability to take a deep breath.

• **Relaxation and stress release.** Holding deep stretches creates relaxation and releases stress. Even mental stress builds muscular tension, which must eventually be released if you are to enjoy good physical health. Remember the discussion of manomaya kosha in chapter 1. Every layer of your being is affected by the other layers. As you hold these poses, monitor your body for tightness and rigidity. At the same time monitor for tight or rigid thoughts, and notice the effect of those thoughts on your muscles. Breathe deeply into tense areas and, as you exhale, consciously work to dissolve the tension. If you notice negative thoughts, replace them with positive thoughts. You should do this mind–body work daily, both on and off your mat.

> For a muscle to lengthen and maintain its new shape, it must be held in a stretch for 30 to 45 seconds. Thus, you should hold every mountain III pose for 5 to 10 breaths, slowing down each inhalation and exhalation so that your body has time to relax and elongate. Just as you must exercise regularly in order to maintain strength and reduce stress, you must stretch often to maintain flexibility. Yoga is a practice to be enjoyed for a lifetime. Remember to listen to your body, relax, and breathe your way into a peaceful space.

**Heat and Flexibility**

Most people think of stretching as a way to increase flexibility and reduce injury. Flexibility is usually defined as the ability to move a joint through its full range of motion (ROM). As a technique to reduce injury, many assume that stretching before exercise or athletic activity helps prepare muscles for movement. However, research cannot confirm that flexibility exercises done before elevation of core body temperature are effective in reducing injury.

Two essential properties of muscles—elasticity and plasticity—allow them to return to their original state after a stretch. If they didn't, the muscles would lengthen continuously until they became so loose that no movement was possible. The plastic properties of muscles allow them to adapt to the continued stress placed on them and to retain those adaptations. If muscles were not plastic, you wouldn't be able strengthen or stretch them; they would remain the same. Both of these qualities—elasticity and plasticity—become more evident when an elevation in core body temperature occurs. Another way of saying this is that muscles improve more rapidly if you work them when they are warm.

Thus, once you have sufficiently elevated your core body temperature, you can begin using movements that condition your body for greater strength, stretch, and flexibility. Your deepest flexibility stretches will occur near the end of your workout, when your body is warmest and your muscles' elasticity and plasticity are optimal.

The increasing popularity of hot yoga needs to be approached with caution. Just because one practices in a heated room does not eliminate the need to warm up the muscles and joints properly. Practicing in a moderately heated room can be very comfortable, but when the heat and humidity are too high, people with certain health conditions can be at risk. If you do choose to practice in the heat, see your doctor or other health care practitioner for advice pertaining to any health conditions you have. Drink plenty of water before, during, and after the practice to stay properly hydrated. Whatever temperature you practice in, follow the YogaFit warm-up and three-mountain format in order to ensure a safe practice. And don't forget to listen to your body.

# Inversions

Inversions are done at the end of mountain III, your cool-down phase. These six inversions are covered in this chapter:

- Legs up the wall
- Shoulderstand

- Plow
- Rabbit
- L-shape forearm balance
- L-shape handstand

In addition to the health benefits already mentioned for the deep stretches, some inversions also increase strength and flexibility, whereas others are extremely relaxing. All inversions prepare your mind and body to let go of tension during final relaxation pose.

The health benefits of being upside down are many. The medical community has begun to realize what yoga practitioners have taught for thousands of years, namely that inversions have a positive impact on your mental and physical well-being. These are some of the benefits of turning upside down:

- You reverse the pull of gravity, allowing venous blood to flow easily back to your heart and lungs for improved circulation.
- You improve blood flow to your brain for a natural pick-me-up and improved concentration.
- You relieve varicose veins and spider veins.
- You reduce your heart rate and blood pressure.
- You boost your immune system.
- You create traction in your spine, removing pressure from the discs between your vertebrae.

**Chronic stress increases your risk of obesity, depression, heart disease, cancer, and many more diseases. One of the culprits in cases of chronic stress is elevated levels of a hormone called cortisol. Although cortisol is useful in circumstances that require immediate energy and action, too much can be harmful. Even just one yoga practice a week can lower your cortisol levels. Deep breathing, deep and relaxing stretches, and a focused mind all help to calm the fight-or-flight response and induce a healing state of relaxation.**

Note that nearly all of the inversions in this chapter (all except legs up the wall) are not recommended for certain conditions, including pregnancy (legs up the wall not recommended after the first trimester), high blood pressure, glaucoma and other eye conditions, neck injury, and cervical arthritis. Ask your doctor which inversions are appropriate for you. In mountains I, II, or III, rest in child's pose and check in with your body.

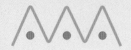

# Child's Pose

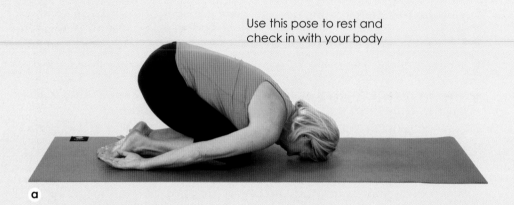

Use this pose to rest and check in with your body

a

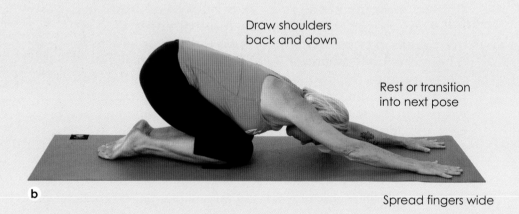

Draw shoulders back and down

Rest or transition into next pose

b

Spread fingers wide

**STRENGTHENS:**
  mind–body connection
**STRETCHES:**
  lower back • gluteal muscles •
  shoulders (extended child's pose)

Child's pose is a mountain I, II, and III pose. To ensure that it is a comfortable position for you to rest and reflect, try both variations of this pose—the wide-knee child's pose and the extended child's pose.

## Getting Into the Pose

Begin kneeling on all fours. Push your hips back to your heels, and bring your arms around to the sides of your body (figure *a*). To stretch your shoulders or to transition to another pose, reach your arms out in front of you for an extended child's pose (figure *b*). To make more room for your body, separate your thighs for a wide-knee version of child's pose.

## Holding the Pose

Rest and breathe, allowing your body to completely relax.

## Modifications

Rest your head on your fists or a block, or your chest on a block for greater back and neck support. If you have knee pain or discomfort, place a rolled-up yoga mat or folded blanket behind your knees.

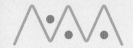

# Kneeling Lunge and Crescent Lunge

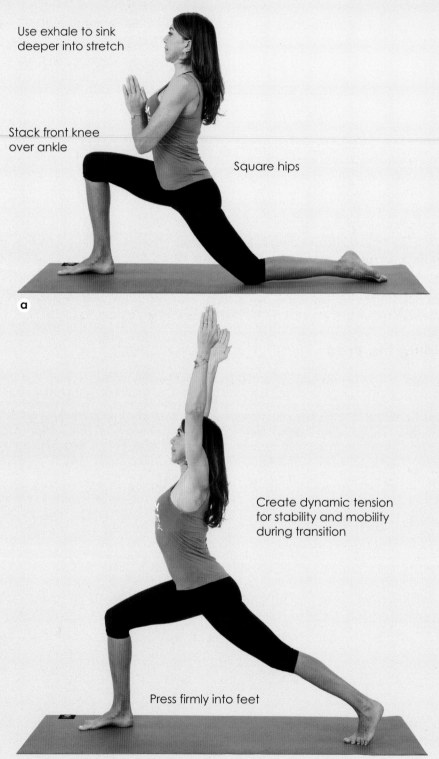

Use exhale to sink deeper into stretch

Stack front knee over ankle

Square hips

**a**

Create dynamic tension for stability and mobility during transition

Press firmly into feet

**b**

Kneeling lunge and crescent lunge open the front of your hips, which tend to tighten after long periods of sitting, running, or cycling. Stretching your hip flexors helps keep you standing upright, preventing low-back problems. Do kneeling lunge and crescent lunge during valley I as part of sun salutations and within your mountain II work.

## Getting Into the Pose

**Kneeling lunge (figure *a*):** From all fours, place one foot forward between your hands, stacking the knee over the ankle.

**Crescent lunge (figure *b*):** Lift your back knee off the floor and straighten your back leg, pressing your back heel toward the wall behind you.

## Holding the Pose

In either pose, face forward and place your hands on your forward thigh or at your chest in prayer position, or raise your arms overhead. Lift the arch of the front foot to create dynamic tension in the legs and core to keep the hips joints supported. Switch sides.

## Modification

In kneeling lunge or crescent lunge, reduce the intensity by placing your fingertips on the floor.

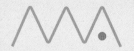

## Quadriceps Stretch

Direct breath into tight muscles

Roll shoulders back and down to open chest

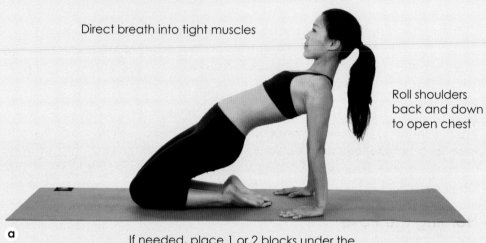

**a**

If needed, place 1 or 2 blocks under the hips for added support for the knees

Explore feeling maximum sensation without pain

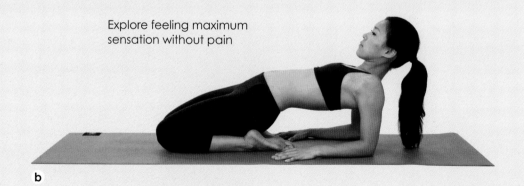

**b**

Although people rely on their quadriceps daily for strength and power, most people tend to stretch them far less than their counterpart, the hamstrings. Use this pose in mountain III to release and lengthen these workhorse muscles.

## Getting Into the Pose

From a kneeling position, sit back on your heels. Place your hands on the floor next to your side. Lift your hips and chest to the sky (figure *a*). For a greater challenge and a deeper stretch, place your forearms on the floor, keeping the heels directly under the hips to protect the knee joints (figure *b*).

## Holding the Pose

In both versions of the pose, increase the stretch by pushing your hips forward and lifting your chest.

## Modifications

If you have a knee injury or discomfort, or if you have tight quadriceps, place a chair, step, or bench behind you for support.

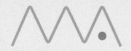

Lift the heart and lengthen the spine to enhance stretch in the hamstrings

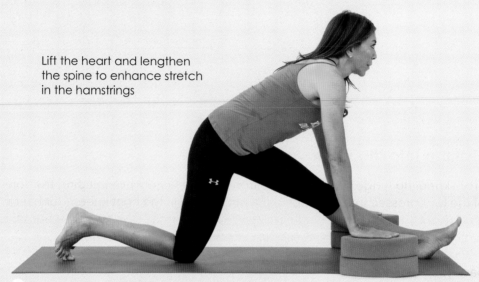

**a**

If needed, place a blanket under the knee

Lift the heart center and relax the shoulders down

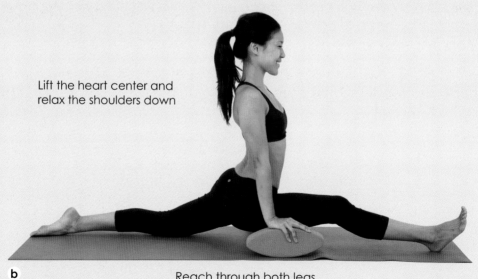

**b**

Reach through both legs and keep the hips forward

Forward splits pose is a mountain III pose helpful for loosening the hips and is especially helpful for runners and cyclists whose hips tend to become tight from the repetitive motion.

## Getting Into the Pose

From kneeling lunge pose, slide the front foot forward while keeping the sole of the foot pressed into the floor and a microbend in the front knee. Your hands are supporting you on the floor or on a block (figure *a*). Engage mula bandha and uddiyana bandha to protect the ligaments in the hips as you slowly lower toward the floor. The front toes can lift off the floor and reach forward as the back toes reach back.

## Holding the Pose

Hands can be kept at the sides of the body (figure *b*) or, for more sensation, sweep them up overhead and hold. Hold the pose for 5 to 10 breaths, and switch sides. To come out of the pose, tuck the back toes under, lifting the kneecap and slowly sliding the front foot back under the knee to lunge.

## Modifications

Use a block (or two chairs) on either side of the hips to create more height if the hips are tight. Only lower as far as you feel comfortable. Keep the front leg bent as needed.

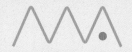

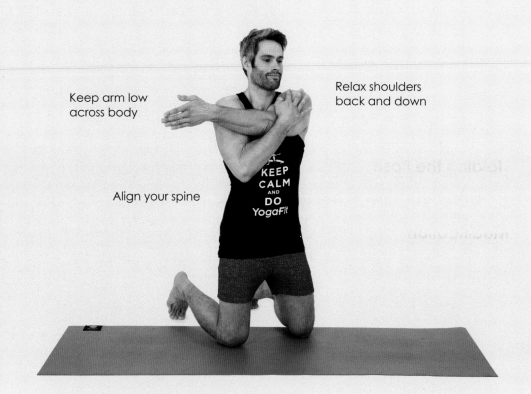

Keep arm low
across body

Relax shoulders
back and down

Align your spine

This pose is helpful for swimmers, weightlifters, and other athletes with tight upper backs and shoulders. Practice it near the beginning of mountain III before you come down onto your back.

## Getting Into the Pose

From a kneeling position, draw one arm low across the front of your body. With your opposite hand, hold your triceps and gently stretch the back of your shoulder.

## Holding the Pose

Sit up tall as you continue gently drawing your arm low across your body.

## Modification

If you have a knee injury or discomfort, practice this pose in an upright seated position.

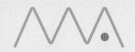

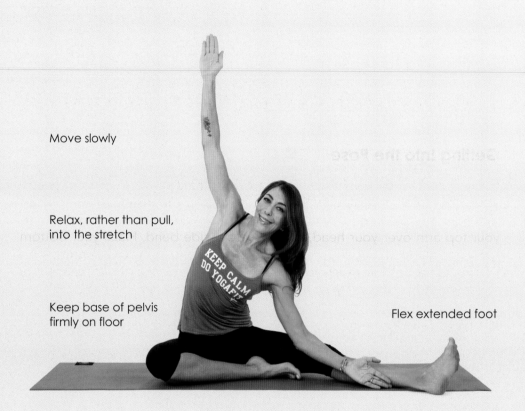

Move slowly

Relax, rather than pull, into the stretch

Keep base of pelvis firmly on floor

Flex extended foot

**STRENGTHENS:**
quads • lower back • oblique abdominal muscles

**STRETCHES:**
hamstrings • hip adductors • chest • shoulders • oblique abdominal muscles

This mountain III pose is a deep stretch for the upper and lower body, and it also strengthens your torso. Come out of this pose slowly and with awareness to protect your back.

## Getting Into the Pose

From seated straddle splits, bend one knee, placing the sole of your foot on your inner thigh. Keeping both sit bones (ischial tuberosities) on the floor, slide your bottom hand down the inside of your leg toward your foot. Reach your top arm over your head, coming into a side bend. Place your bottom hand on your extended leg, or grab the outside edge of your extended foot. Roll your chest as you reach your top arm to the sky. For a greater challenge, lower your top arm over your ear, reaching for your extended foot.

## Holding the Pose

Continue opening your chest while drawing your shoulder blades down your back. Firm your quadriceps to help release your hamstrings. Switch sides.

## Modifications

If you have a knee injury or discomfort, keep both legs extended in seated straddle splits. If you're unable to reach your extended foot with your bottom hand, use a strap.

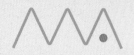

Relax the head down toward the knee and inhale, directing the breath into the upper back

Draw your navel toward the spine firmly as you exhale

Push through the heel

Use a strap if hands do not connect

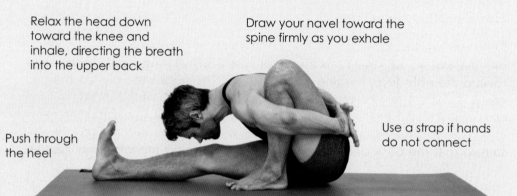

**STRETCHES:**
hamstrings • gluteal muscles •
upper back • lower back •
shoulders

Sage pose is a complex mountain III pose that provides a wonderful relaxing stretch for the upper back and shoulders, the low back, and the hamstrings. The breath is instrumental in deepening the sensations in this pose.

## Getting Into the Pose

From a seated position, bend the left knee and plant the left foot firmly on the mat, but let the knee relax away from the body slightly. Reach both hands toward the right foot, hinging from the hips. The right knee can be bent as needed. Take a few breaths here, reaching the center of the chest forward with each exhalation. Next, reach the left hand backward, turning the palm outward. Continue reaching backward as you wrap your arm around the left shin so that the back of the left hand is now touching the left hip or gluteal muscles. Reach the right hand around the opposite side to the back, reaching toward the left hand. Hands can clasp together if they touch, or you can hold onto the waistband. Relax into the pose by flexing the spine and dropping the head.

## Holding the Pose

Breathe into the space behind the chest to deepen the sensation. Hold for 5 to 10 breaths, and repeat on the other side.

## Modifications

If your hands don't touch, use a strap. Set a strap on the floor in the shape of a U with the ends toward the front. As you sweep your arms around, pick up the strap on each side and begin to walk the hands toward one another as far as you feel comfortable. If the hamstrings are tight, bend the straight leg.

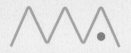

Focus on rest and relaxation

Keep spine neutral and
abdominals warm

Practice sinking
breath

Gently push hips back

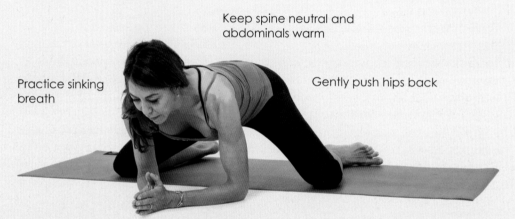

Make sure your body is
thoroughly warm

Try frog pose in mountain III to stretch tight inner thigh muscles after the demanding strength work you do for your legs in mountain II. Succumb to gravity in this pose for total body relaxation.

## Getting Into the Pose

Begin kneeling, facing the long edge of your mat. Separate your knees out wide to each side, keeping your ankles directly behind your knees and your feet flexed. Slowly lower your upper body toward the floor.

## Holding the Pose

Gently push your hips back, keeping your spine neutral and abdominal muscles firm. Use sinking breath technique (see chapter 3) to help release muscular tension.

## Modifications

For knee injuries or discomfort, use a wide-knee child's pose or a dead bug pose.

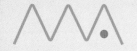

Practice sinking breath

Draw forward using
abdominals

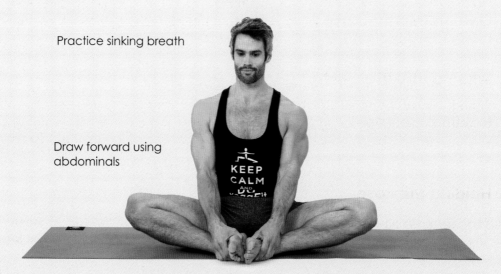

Avoid pulling feet

Do butterfly pose during mountain III after your body is warm. This pose is a favorite among athletes with tight hips and inner thighs, such as bikers and runners, as well as people who sit in a chair for long periods.

## Getting Into the Pose

Sitting tall with a straight spine, place the soles of your feet together in front of you. Use your outer thighs to draw your knees toward the floor. Holding your ankles, reach your chest forward as far as you can before releasing into the fold.

## Holding the Pose

Keeping your elbows back along your body, continue to draw your knees toward the floor. Use sinking breath (see chapter 3) to help release muscle tension.

## Modification

If you are unable to maintain a straight spine, sit on a rolled-up yoga mat or folded blanket.

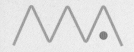

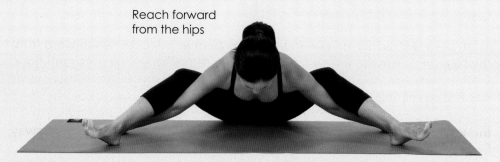

Reach forward from the hips

Draw abdominals in toward spine, and exhale slowly to relax more deeply

Turtle pose in mountain III gives you an option when you want to increase the stretch of deeper muscles in the back and hips. You use the activity of the legs and the arms to bring yourself into a deeper forward flexion.

## Getting Into the Pose

From seated straddle splits with the knees bent as needed, flex forward from the hips and slide the arms under the upper legs with the palms to the floor. Create dynamic tension in the arms and shoulders by pressing the fingers and mounds at the base of the fingers into the mat (activating hasta bandha), and press the upper arms into the backs of the legs as you also begin to extend the knee joint and move toward a straighter leg. Draw the shoulders away from the ears, and reach the center of the chest forward.

## Holding the Pose

Contract the abdominal muscles to assist in relaxing the back muscles. Take a deep breath in, lifting slightly, and then exhale as you sink a little deeper. Follow this pose with incline plank or simply lie on your back for a few breaths.

## Modifications

Bend the knees if the hamstrings are tight. To protect your shoulders, use caution when pressing the legs into the arms. Be mindful to always move with your breath, and use dynamic tension to keep the joints stable when applying pressure.

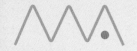

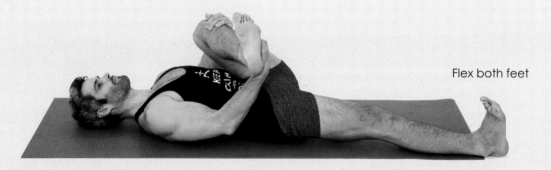

Direct breath into
tight hip muscles

Flex both feet

Upside-down pigeon pose is a deep stretch that releases your hips, where you store much of your tension and stress. Releasing this area allows you to experience more agility and balance in your body and mind. Because you do this pose on your back, completely supported by gravity, it also restores and relaxes your spine. Use this pose near the end of mountain III, before you begin inversions.

## Getting Into the Pose

From your back, lift your left foot off the floor and place your left ankle across your abdomen, flexing both feet. Hold your left shin with both hands, and gently draw your left knee toward your chest until you feel a stretch in your right hip.

## Holding the Pose

With each exhalation, continue drawing your knee close, focusing on releasing your right hip. Switch sides.

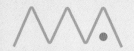

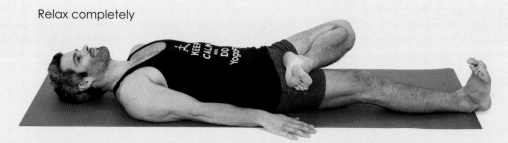

Move slowly and listen to your body

Relax completely

Place foot anywhere on leg
that is comfortable

Because you're on your back, supine half lotus pose allows your entire body to relax. For this reason, it's particularly beneficial near the end of mountain III.

## Getting Into the Pose

From your back, place one foot on your opposite thigh near the top of your leg. Allow the knee of your bent leg to relax toward the floor. Proceed carefully and with great awareness, without forcing your knee into the pose.

## Holding the Pose

Monitor your body for any sign of tension or resistance. With every exhalation, release this tension. Switch sides.

## Modification

If you have knee pain or discomfort, do upside-down pigeon pose instead.

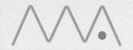

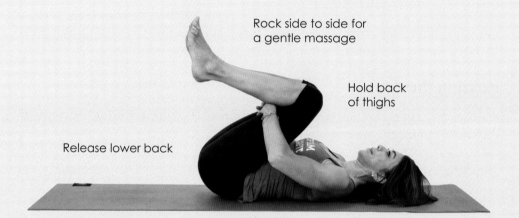

Rock side to side for a gentle massage

Hold back of thighs

Release lower back

Similar to child's pose, knees to chest pose is a restorative, restful place to return to any time during mountain III that you need a break. Also use this pose following backbends to release your low back and neutralize your spine.

## Getting Into the Pose

Lie down with your back on the floor. Bring your knees into your chest. Hold onto the backs of your thighs.

## Holding the Pose

Keep drawing your knees toward your chest while keeping your tailbone on the floor. For a gentle back massage, rock side to side.

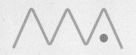

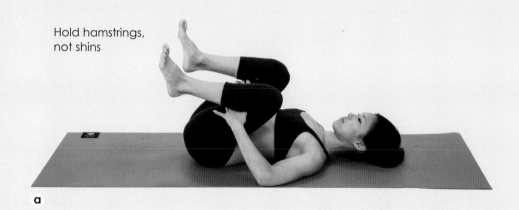

Hold hamstrings, not shins

a

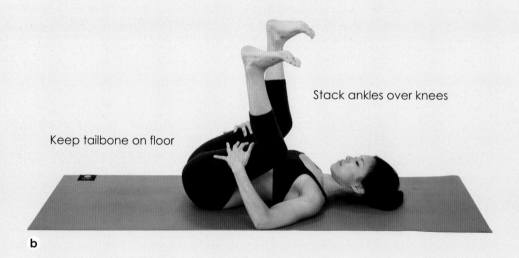

Stack ankles over knees

Keep tailbone on floor

b

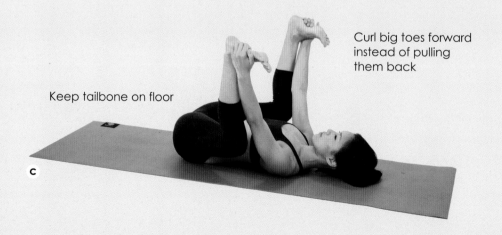

Curl big toes forward instead of pulling them back

Keep tailbone on floor

c

Practice this pose near the end of mountain III, before you begin inversions.

## Getting Into the Pose

From knees to chest pose, hold your hamstrings and draw your knees down toward the floor (figure *a*). When your tailbone is resting on the floor and your thighs are pulled in next to the rib cage, pause to breathe deeply, feeling the rib cage press into the thighs. Then lift the soles of your feet toward the sky, so that the ankles stack over the knees (figure *b*). For a greater challenge, grab the bottom of your feet and draw your knees toward the floor while bringing your elbows out to each side (figure *c*). Keep your ankles stacked over your knees and your tailbone and shoulders pressed to the floor.

## Holding the Pose

In all versions of this pose, continue drawing your knees toward the floor. Rest your head, shoulders, and tailbone on the floor as you stretch. Allow yourself to feel supported by gravity as you release physical and emotional tension from your back and hips.

## Modifications

If this pose is uncomfortable, stay in the knees to chest pose. If your tailbone lifts off the floor, keep your knees bent, as shown in figure *a*.

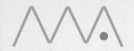

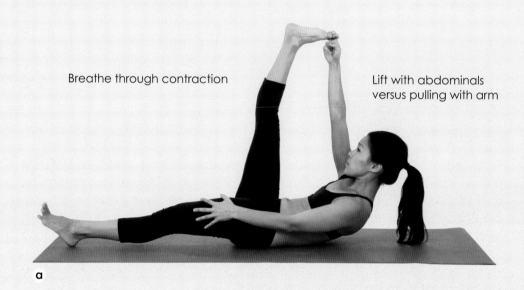

Breathe through contraction

Lift with abdominals versus pulling with arm

a

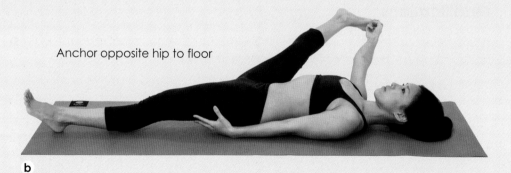

Relax and breathe deeply

Anchor opposite hip to floor

b

**STRENGTHENS:**
 abdominals • hip flexors
**STRETCHES:**
 gluteal muscles • hip adductors •
 hamstrings

This two-for-one pose strengthens your abdominal muscles while increasing flexibility in your legs. Do this pose during mountain III.

## Getting Into the Pose

From your back, lift your right leg. Grab your big toe with the index and middle fingers of your right hand, and place your left hand on your left thigh. Exhale, lifting your forehead toward your knee, and hold for five breaths while concentrating on your abdominal muscles contracting strongly (figure *a*). Inhaling, release your head back to the floor as you open your leg to the same side (figure *b*). Look over your opposite shoulder, and hold for five breaths. Inhale, again lifting your leg back to center and your forehead toward your knee; hold for five breaths. Release, and switch sides.

## Holding the Pose

When your leg is extended to the side, keep both hips on the floor. Press through your heels, and straighten your legs.

## Modifications

If you have tight hamstrings, use a strap across the ball of your foot, or keep your knee bent throughout each phase of the pose.

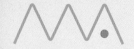

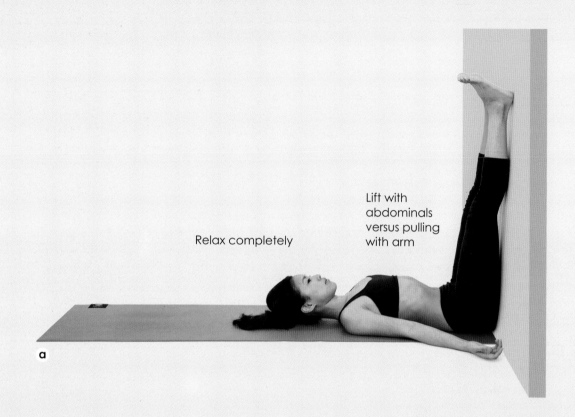

Relax completely

Lift with abdominals versus pulling with arm

a

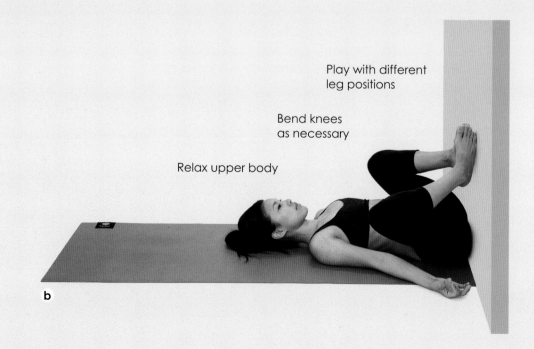

Play with different leg positions

Bend knees as necessary

Relax upper body

b

In this mountain III inversion, it's hard not to relax. To add a deep, relaxing stretch, experiment with various leg positions, such as straddle splits or a pose similar to butterfly pose, in which the soles of your feet are together and your knees are open. Remember to check with your doctor before doing any inversions.

## Getting Into the Pose

From knees to chest pose, roll over onto one side until your gluteal muscles touch the wall. Use your hands to roll onto your back, straightening your legs up the wall (figure *a*).

## Holding the Pose

Separate your legs slightly to breathe more easily into the bottom of your lungs (figure *b*).

## Modification

Without a wall available, make fists and place them under your hips for support.

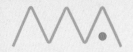

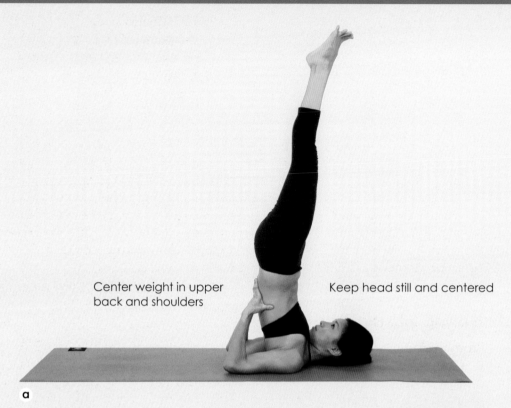

Center weight in upper back and shoulders

Keep head still and centered

**a**

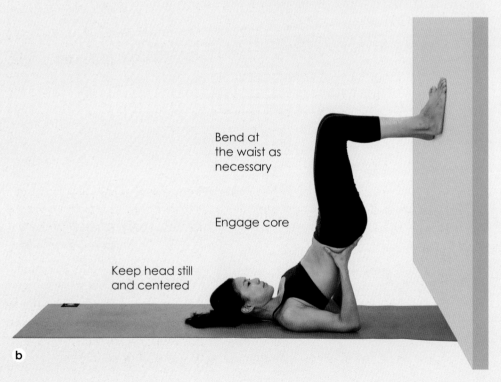

Bend at the waist as necessary

Engage core

Keep head still and centered

**b**

Shoulderstand is an inversion that can potentially create compression in the neck, so special attention moving into and out of this pose is a must! YogaFit teaches moving into shoulderstand from bridge pose or legs up the wall for additional support, noting that you can choose to stay with your feet on the wall as shown in figure b. Shoulderstand requires a significant amount of opening in the chest and shoulders to be able to keep the cervical spine safe. This pose is believed to stimulate the thyroid gland, increasing your metabolism. Again, remember to ask your doctor which inversions are appropriate for you before you try them.

## Getting Into the Pose

From bridge pose, make sure no part of your spine is on the mat (see SPA 5: relax the shoulders back and down), walk your feet toward your shoulders to bring your hands to your hips, and support the low back. Using your abdominal muscles, lift one knee toward the nose followed by the other, straightening your legs and lifting your hips as high as comfortable (figure a). For the safety of your cervical spine, do not move your head or neck. For less pressure on your neck, keep a slight bend at the waist; again, don't move your head or neck.

From legs up the wall: Bend your knees so that your feet are flat on the wall. Walking the shoulder blades toward the spine and pressing the feet firmly into the wall, lift the hips until they are stacked over the shoulders (figure b), placing the hands behind the hips for more support. Keep the feet on the wall, or practice lifting one leg off the wall then the other for gradual strengthening.

## Holding the Pose

Breathe into and through your throat and chest. Always follow with knees to chest pose. If desired, move to plow pose, then come out of the pose by rolling into a knees to chest pose, using the abdominal muscles to brake the movement.

## Modifications

Remember, both shoulderstand and plow require the shoulders and chest to be open. Shoulderstand and plow pose are not recommended for people with neck or back issues and with certain medical conditions. As an alternative, and with your doctor's permission, practice legs up the wall pose instead.

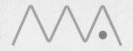

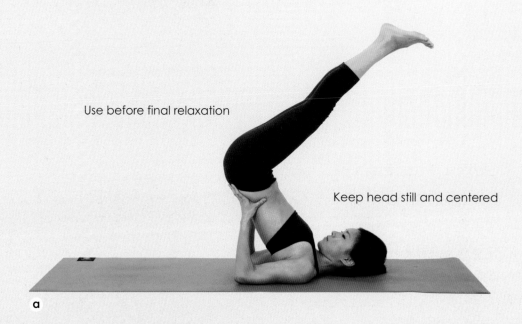

Use before final relaxation

Keep head still and centered

a

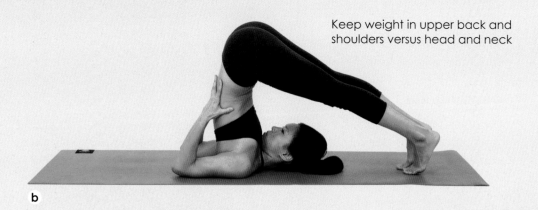

Keep weight in upper back and shoulders versus head and neck

b

**STRENGTHENS:**
  abdominal muscles
**STRETCHES:**
  gluteal muscles • lower back •
  hamstrings

Plow pose is most effective in mountain III near the end of your session, when your body is thoroughly warm. Because plow pose compresses the throat, it is believed to stimulate the thyroid gland, increasing metabolism. Remember to ask your doctor which inversions are appropriate for you.

## Getting Into the Pose

From shoulderstand, support your lower back with your hands (figure *a*) as you slowly straighten your legs and place your toes on the floor (figure *b*).

## Holding the Pose

Keep your legs straight. If your feet don't touch the floor, support your lower back with your hands. Breathe into your throat. Come out of the pose by moving back into half or full shoulderstand, and roll slowly back down into a knees to chest pose using the abdominal muscles to brake the movement.

## Modifications

As mentioned at the start of the chapter, plow pose is not recommended for people with certain medical conditions. As an alternative, and with your doctor's permission, practice legs up the wall pose instead. If your toes don't reach the floor in plow pose, place the tops of your feet on a chair.

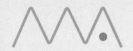

## Fish

Check in with your body

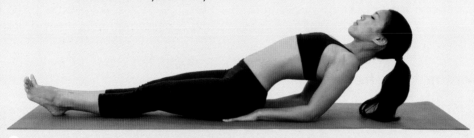

**a**

Practice expanding breath

Bring legs together

Open throat without
dropping head back

Point toes

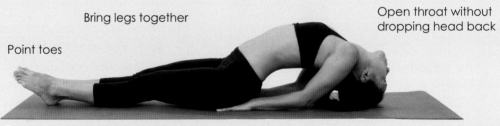

**b**

Fish pose is an effective counterpose when practiced directly after the plow and shoulderstand at the end of mountain III. This pose can alleviate certain chest disorders and promote a healthy heart. The pose might also stimulate the thyroid, increasing metabolism.

## Getting Into the Pose

From plow pose or shoulderstand, bring your knees to your chest. Extend your legs along the floor, and slide your hands under your hips, palms down (figure *a*). Bring your elbows toward each other beneath your back. Point your toes toward the floor as you reach back in the opposite direction with the crown of your head, shifting your body back slightly as well (figure *b*).

## Holding the Pose

Lift your chest, and rest your head lightly on the floor, maintaining space in the back of your neck; relax. Your breath should feel deep and easy; if it doesn't, adjust your position. Always follow fish pose with knees to chest pose.

## Modification

As necessary, place a rolled-up yoga mat or blanket under your upper back for cushion and support.

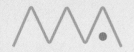

Lift the hips to find more
stretch through the back

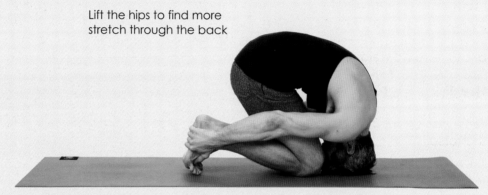

Do not place
weight on
the head

This mountain III pose is an inversion option for those that want the benefits of an inversion without any pressure on the cervical vertebrae.

## Getting Into the Pose

From child's pose, curl the toes under. Reaching your arms back, wrap your palms around the soles of the feet. Tuck your chin into your chest, and lift your hips away from your feet. The top of your head will be grazing the mat, but there is *no* weight on the head.

## Holding the Pose

Taking deep, full breaths into the upper back, imagine creating space inside the torso.

## Modifications

Use a strap around the feet if your arms don't reach back far enough to hold the feet.

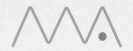

## L-Shaped Handstand

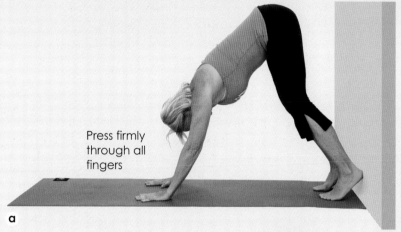

Press firmly through all fingers

Press heels into wall

a

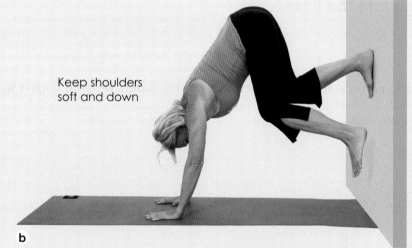

Keep shoulders soft and down

Press feet firmly into wall and engage core as you walk feet up wall

b

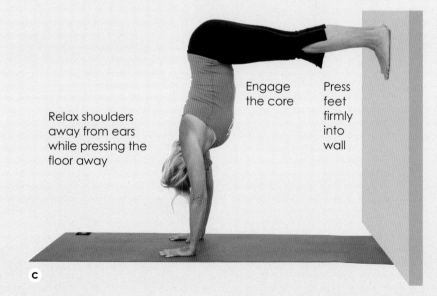

Relax shoulders away from ears while pressing the floor away

Engage the core

Press feet firmly into wall

c

The next two poses are helpful in progressing your practice to include hand-stands, forearm balance, and eventually scorpion. Use the wall as support while you get used to being upside down (which can be scary), and gradually build up strength in the upper body. Learning to trust your upper body strength will happen gradually, so have fun with these poses and appreciate the wall as a friend!

## Getting Into the Pose

From downward-facing dog with your heels pressed against a sturdy wall (figure a), activate your core and begin to walk slowly up the wall until your feet reach hip level. Press the feet firmly into the wall, and activate pada bandha. The hands should be stacked directly under the shoulders with the fingers spread wide (starfish hands; figure b). If you find your hands in front of the shoulders, walk the feet down and reposition them closer to the wall.

## Holding the Pose

Press your fingers firmly into the mat, and press the feet into the wall for a fully active core. Draw the energy from the arms and the legs to the center of the body (figure c). For more sensation lift one leg off the wall, and reach the heel toward the sky. Switch sides. Concentrate on a slow, steady breath. Follow with child's pose.

## Modifications

If you need to minimize pressure on the wrists, then try forearm balance instead. If your feet slide down the wall, then concentrate more on core activation by drawing the muscles of the pelvic floor up toward the heart.

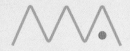

# L-Shaped Forearm Balance

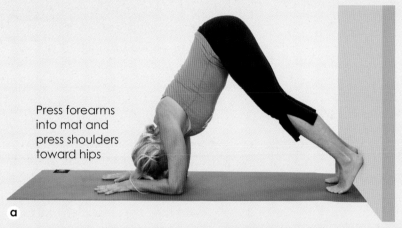

Press forearms into mat and press shoulders toward hips

Press heels firmly into wall

a

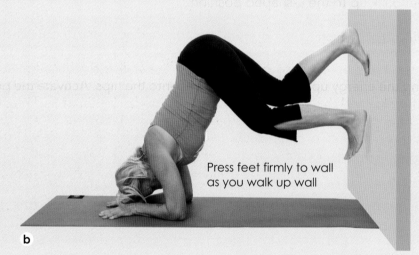

Press feet firmly to wall as you walk up wall

b

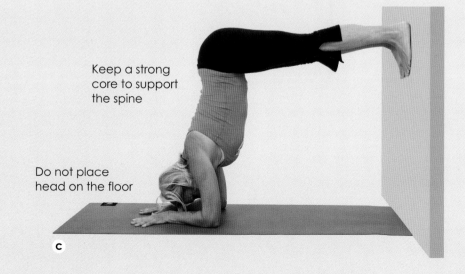

Keep a strong core to support the spine

Do not place head on the floor

c

## Getting Into the Pose

From dolphin pose with the feet flat against the wall, elbows shoulder width apart and forearms and palms pressing into the floor (figure *a*), lift the hips and walk the feet up the wall to hip level. The shoulders should be stacked directly over the elbows (figure *b*). If the elbows are in front of the shoulders, walk the feet back down, reposition the elbows closer to the wall, and walk the feet back up to the L-shaped position.

## Holding the Pose

Activate the core by pressing the feet into the wall and lifting the arches, drawing the energy up through the legs and into the hips. Activate the pelvic floor muscles and the transverse abdominal muscles by drawing the energy toward the center of the body and upward toward the center of your chest. Reach the heart center toward the fingers, and keep the head in line with the spine (figure *c*). For more sensation, lift one leg off the wall and press the heel toward the sky. Switch sides. Maintain a slow, deep breath. Follow with child's pose.

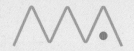
Stay present in the moment

Breathe naturally

Relax completely

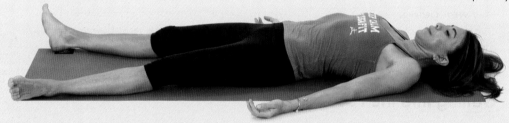

At the end of a YogaFit session, you have completed your work*out* and prepared your mind and body for your work *in*. You should never confuse activity with productivity. This statement is particularly true in final relaxation pose. This is the one pose in which you are instructed to do nothing, and yet you receive a lot.

Final relaxation pose allows you an opportunity to again become aware of your body and mind, mentally and physically integrating the benefits of your practice. It also provides an important transition back into your daily routine. Finally, this pose helps release muscular tension and stress for improved health and well-being.

Final relaxation pose is an integral part of any yoga practice and should never be rushed or skipped. At the end of mountain III, allow 6 to 10 minutes for final relaxation.

## Getting Into the Pose

Lie on your back (or in any position that allows you total comfort and relaxation). Turn your palms toward the sky, and allow your feet to roll open.

## Holding the Pose

Let your breath return to its natural, rhythmic cycle. Continue to release stress and tension, finding peace and calm.

## Modifications

For low-back discomfort, place your feet flat on the floor and bend your knees, allowing them to lean against one another. For added comfort, place a pillow or towel behind your knees or your head.

PART III

# Putting It All Together

CHAPTER  10

# Workouts for Fitness and Sports

 A regular YogaFit practice will help you in your sports and fitness whether you are a weekend athlete, a competitive athlete, or just want to move more comfortably and reduce chances of injury.

In this chapter several YogaFit workouts are presented to choose from, depending on your familiarity with yoga and exercise in general. Beginning your YogaFit practice is a matter of choosing to begin to consciously breathe, and then you can simply think of adding movements that you coordinate with the breath. If you are new to yoga, start with the beginning YogaFit practice or, simply, one of the warm ups. In the workouts you'll work all your body parts, including your legs, arms, torso, sides, shoulders, neck, back, abdominal muscles, and inner organs. Each workout combines standing poses with seated and lying-down poses, and progresses from a warm-up with heat-building sequences to deep, relaxing stretches and a cool-down. Each pose in each workout is followed by an appropriate counterpose (e.g., a backbend is followed by a forward bend) to keep your body tuned and balanced.

Sometimes you might need to modify or omit poses that are not recommended or appropriate for you because of a medical condition, or if they feel uncomfortable. Be cautious with special conditions such as injuries or pregnancy. Before you begin a workout, review Special Considerations for YogaFit in chapter 2. Also remember to consult your doctor before starting any new workout, including the YogaFit workouts. You might occasionally feel sensations that are mildly uncomfortable as your body adjusts to a new workout or pose, and this is fine, but if the discomfort turns to pain, cease the workout or pose immediately. Don't wait to adjust to the pain or for the pain to subside. Finally, allow yourself to rest when you need to. Do what you need to do to enjoy your workout session; enjoyment will keep you coming back.

# Before You Start

As you learned in part I, a successful YogaFit practice is more than a work-out—it's an experience for the mind and body that leads to greater health and joy. But to realize these benefits, you need to prepare yourself adequately and remember that yoga is more about the journey than the destination. Each time you step on your mat, be prepared to listen to your body and drop any expectations you may have for that day's practice. Savor the uniqueness of each practice! These key points should help you move in the right direction:

• **Familiarize yourself with the poses.** Take time to get familiar with the poses described in part II. The format of the workouts in this chapter are designed to help you remember how to do the poses, but full descriptions of the poses and their modifications are not included here. It's one thing to know the names of the poses and how they're supposed to look; it's another to understand how to make them fit your body and how to safely transition from one to the next.

• **Move consciously and with control from pose to pose.** When per-forming a workout, observe your body without judgment, realizing that each body has its limits. When you need a break, move into child's pose for a few breaths. Listen to your body; only you know what is good for you on any given day. Also, understand that your body will be tight in certain areas and more flexible in others. One side of your body will be more flexible than the other, and one side of your body will be stronger than the other. Observe and learn. Over time your YogaFit sessions should help you even out imbalances.

• **Be patient and consistent.** Often, you can accomplish certain poses only after practicing them regularly for a while. One of the beautiful moments in yoga is when you find yourself in a pose that you could not do in previous workouts. But never force a pose. Never push yourself beyond your limits.

YogaFit is best practiced three to five times a week for 30 to 60 minutes each session. Make time for your routine, and you'll soon notice a difference in the way you feel. You'll also learn that there is no "bad" or "wrong" YogaFit practice as long as you go at your own pace, breathe effectively, and allow yourself to experience how each pose feels at each moment. Remember, any movement is good movement as long as it is safe movement.

• **Learn that each practice is a reward in itself.** Give yourself permis-sion to explore yourself and your practice with each session. If you see each YogaFit session as new and unique, you'll feel better without the risk of burning out or getting bored. Remember the YogaFit essence *Let go of your expectations* each time you come to your mat. Find new ways to express each pose as well as new ways to enter into and exit out of each pose safely. If you do, you'll be grateful for any shift or improvement, and you'll never leave your mat disappointed or feeling that you wasted your time. Make YogaFit your companion for life. It can help you achieve all your goals, not just the physical ones.

# YogaFit Workouts

The following workouts vary in length and level of difficulty. Some are for beginners, and others for people who have experience with YogaFit or who are in excellent physical condition. Four kinds of workouts are presented here:

- **Beginning YogaFit**—This short, less-intense workout for beginning students can be modified easily for special conditions. Those with more experience may come back to beginning YogaFit when they need a restorative or healing practice session.

- **Flex and Flow**—This is a slightly longer beginner to intermediate workout that combines repetitive movement with static holds. It's a great total body workout that will make you sweat.

- **YogaCore**—Ready for a challenge? This longer workout targets your midsection, including your gluteal muscles and low back, for muscular power and stamina. You'll do plenty of stretching and balance work as well.

- **Power YogaFit**—This workout is the most physically demanding offered, with more complex sequences and additional flow series to increase heat and intensity. This workout is for healthy and experienced people looking to take their physical practice to the next level.

No matter what your experience or fitness level, start with the Beginning YogaFit workout to familiarize yourself with YogaFit and introduce your body and mind to the new format. Afterward, experiment with the other three workouts until you find one in which you feel challenged, yet successful. Stick with one, or vary your workout regularly, depending on what you need personally and physically. Following the workouts, the section called Taking Your Workout to the Next Level shows you how to progress by altering your workouts so that you always have a place to go as you improve and desire more from each practice.

## Warm-Up

As you learned in chapter 4, a YogaFit session is based on the three mountains format and includes a warm-up, workout, and cool-down. This format ensures effective, safe, and consistent progression in every YogaFit workout. Just as it is important for the workout as a whole to be balanced, it is important for the warm-up be balanced. By targeting every major muscle group in your warm-up and moving the joints through their natural range of motion, you prepare your body to move into the workout phase of mountain II.

Use one of these two balanced, comprehensive warm-ups to prepare for mountain II. The first begins lying down and is effective for beginners, evening workouts, or even midday workouts when your mind is wandering and you need extra help centering. The second warm-up begins standing up—a great way to start the day or to begin a more vigorous practice.

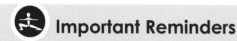

## Important Reminders

- Sun salutations and modified sun salutations are the series of 12 poses described in chapter 4. This series can be done on or off the knees, depending on your strength and stability. In the following workouts, warm up in valley I with the modified version first, then progress to the full version as appropriate for your body, performing two to four sets (or more as your strength and fitness level increase).

- The flow series, or the bottom half of sun salutations, can be done on or off the knees, depending on your strength and stability.

- When you start any series it is easier to start with the same foot, but as you become more comfortable, vary which foot you start with. It is good for your brain to change up the order and how you do things. Repeat each series on the opposite side before moving on.

- As mentioned in chapter 7, to protect the back, the swan dive (see figures *a-c*) and reverse swan dive (see figures *d-f*) are always the transitions between standing forward fold and upright standing poses in workouts or series. Keep your knees bent, spine straight, and arms out to the side as you go either up or down. Avoid reaching directly forward with your arms, because it increases the lever length and might strain your low back (see SPA 7 in chapter 2).

- Always begin with 3 to 5 minutes of deep breathing, then maintain a deep breath throughout, until final relaxation.

- Breathing techniques and locks (see chapter 3) can be added where appropriate.

- Rest when you need to. Generally people take child's pose when resting, but you may use any pose that feels right to you.

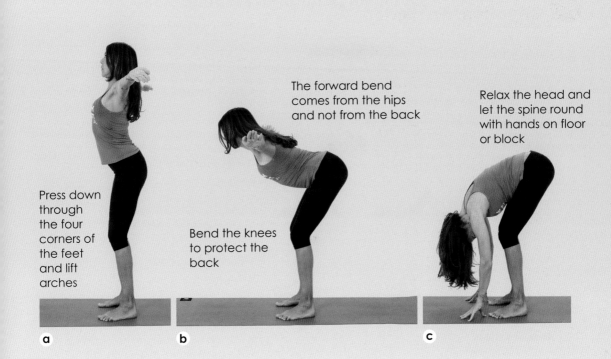

Press down through the four corners of the feet and lift arches

a

The forward bend comes from the hips and not from the back

Bend the knees to protect the back

b

Relax the head and let the spine round with hands on floor or block

c

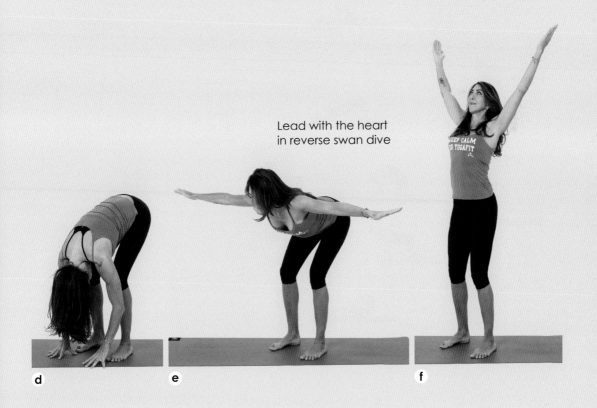

Lead with the heart in reverse swan dive

d

e

f

# Standard Lying-Down Warm-Up

| | | | |
|---|---|---|---|
| **Relaxation on back** (same as final relaxation) | | • 3-5 minutes of deep breathing. | Page 228 |
| **Knees to chest** | | • Hold the back of one thigh, and extend one leg at a time above the mat. Alternate legs.<br>• Repeat 5-10 times, flowing with your breath. | Page 208 |
| **Bridge** | | • Repeat 2-3 times, flowing with your breath.<br>• Inhale as you lift; exhale as you lower your back to the mat. | Page 154 |
| **Ab work** | | • Repeat 5-6 times. | Page 56 |
| **Knees to chest** | | • For a modification, hold the back of one thigh, and extend one leg at a time above the mat. Alternate legs.<br>• Repeat 5-10 times, flowing with your breath. | Page 208 |
| **Flowing bridge** | | • Inhale as you lift; exhale as you lower your back to the mat.<br>• Repeat 2-3 times, flowing with your breath. | Page 154 |
| **Cat and cow** | | • Repeat 5-10 times. | Page 142 |
| **Spinal balance** | | • Repeat 5-10 times. | Page 58 |
| **Child's pose** | | • Pause to check in. | Page 184 |

| Modified flow series | Repeat 5-10 times. Omit cobra; instead push straight back into child's pose from kneeling plank. | | |
|---|---|---|---|
| 1. Child's pose | | • Sink hips toward heels. | Page 184 |
| 2. Kneeling plank | | • Draw forward with a neutral spine. | Page 42 |
| 3. Kneeling crocodile | | • Lower your upper body while lifting your abdominals. | Page 44 |
| 4. Child's pose | | • Draw back, moving from your core. | Page 184 |

## Standard Standing Warm-Up

| Mountain pose | | • 3-5 minutes of deep breathing. | Page 72 |
|---|---|---|---|
| Moonflowers | | • Repeat 5-10 times. | Page 74 |
| Sunflowers | | • Repeat 5-10 times. | Page 76 |
| Chair flow | | • Inhale with arms overhead; exhale sitting back into chair pose.<br>• Repeat 5 or more times. | Page 94 |

> continued

| Swan dive and reverse swan dive | | • Bend the knees and hinge from the hips, bringing the hands to the floor. Reverse the swan dive by bending the knees and returning to mountain pose with a straight spine.<br>• Keep the arms out to the sides, not reaching forward.<br>• Repeat 5 or more times. | Page 236 |
|---|---|---|---|
| | *and* | | |
| Downward-facing dog | | • Repeat 10 times with alternating heel press. | Page 122 |
| Child's pose | | • Hold for 5 breaths. | Page 184 |
| Cat and cow | | • Repeat 10-15 times. | Page 142 |
| Spinal balance | | • Repeat 10-15 times. | Page 58 |
| **Modified flow series** | **Repeat 5-10 times.**<br>**Omit cobra; instead push straight back into child's pose from kneeling plank.** | | |
| *1. Child's pose* | | • Sink hips toward heels. | Page 184 |
| *2. Kneeling plank* | | • Draw forward with a neutral spine. | Page 42 |
| *3. Kneeling crocodile* | | • Lower upper body while lifting abdominals. | Page 44 |
| *4. Child's pose* | | • Draw back, moving from the core. | Page 184 |

| Downward-facing dog | | • Hold for 5 breaths. | Page 122 |
|---|---|---|---|
| Reverse swan dive to mountain pose | | • Bend knees, and return to mountain pose with a straight spine.<br>• Keep arms out to the sides, not reaching forward. | Pages 236 and 72 |

## Beginning YogaFit

Beginning YogaFit is a fluid 45-minute total body workout appropriate for most healthy beginners of any age. Beginning YogaFit is a great place to learn the elements if you are new to yoga.

| MOUNTAIN I: Warm-up | | | |
|---|---|---|---|
| **Standard lying-down warm-up** | | | |
| VALLEY I: Sun salutations | | | |
| **Sun salutations** | **Repeat 2-4 times.** | | |
| 1. Mountain pose | | • Stand with feet hip-width apart.<br>• Establish a strong base | Page 72 |
| 2. Standing forward fold | | • Swan dive into the pose.<br>• Place hands firmly on floor. | Page 120 |

> *continued*

| | VALLEY I: Sun salutations | | |
|---|---|---|---|
| 3. Crescent lunge or kneeling lunge | or | • Reach back with one foot, maintaining alignment with hip. | Page 186 |
| 4. Downward-facing dog or child's pose | or | • Press back, hinging from the hips. | Pages 122 and 184 |
| 5. Plank or kneeling plank | or | • Draw forward with a neutral spine. | Page 42 |
| 6. Crocodile or kneeling crocodile | or | • Lower upper body while lifting abdominals muscles. | Page 44 |
| 7. Upward-facing dog or cobra | or | • Lift and open the chest.<br>• Lengthen out of lower back. | Pages 48 and 46 |
| 8. Downward-facing dog or child's pose | or | • Press back, hinging from the hips. | Pages 122 and 184 |
| 9. Crescent lunge or kneeling lunge | or | • Step forward, stacking knee over ankle. | Page 186 |
| 10. Standing forward fold | | • Engage core.<br>• Use reverse swan dive to return to mountain. | Page 120 |
| 11. Mountain pose | | • Check in with your body and breath. | Page 72 |

| VALLEY I:  Sun salutations | | | |
|---|---|---|---|
| *12. Chair* | | • Relax shoulders back and down.<br>• Keep elbows soft.<br>• Sit back, shifting weight to heels. | Page 94 |

| MOUNTAIN II:  Work | | | |
|---|---|---|---|
| **Hold poses for 3-5 breaths unless otherwise noted.** | | | |
| **Standing lateral flexion** | | • Repeat on both sides. | Page 80 |
| **Standing chest expansion with forward fold** | | • For lower back discomfort or injury, remain standing upright. | Page 130 |
| **Warrior Series** | **Repeat series on both sides.** | | |
| *1. Warrior I* | | • Press back foot flat to floor.<br>• Square shoulders with front of mat.<br>• Engage the core by pressing through the feet and lifting the spine. | Page 82 |
| *2. Warrior II* | | • Face long edge of mat.<br>• Stack forward knee over ankle. | Page 84 |
| *3. Triangle* | | • Maintain neutral spine. | Page 88 |
| *4. Mountain pose* | | • Check in with your body and breath. | Page 72 |

> *continued*

| VALLEY II: Upright standing balance | | | |
|---|---|---|---|
| Tree | | • Hold for 5-10 breaths.<br>• Switch sides. | Page 104 |

| MOUNTAIN III: Cool-Down | | | |
|---|---|---|---|
| **Hold poses for 5-10 breaths unless otherwise noted.** | | | |
| Rabbit and kneeling shoulder stretch | *and* | • Sink hips toward heels. | Pages 222 and 192 |
| Seated straddle splits | | • Point knees and toes up.<br>• Practice sinking breath. | Page 140 |
| Butterfly | | • Soften toward floor.<br>• Avoid pulling feet.<br>• Practice sinking breath. | Page 200 |
| Tabletop | | • Roll shoulders back and down before lifting.<br>• Stack joints. | Page 52 |
| Knees to chest | | • Soften and relax. | Page 208 |
| Dead bug | | • Keep tailbone on floor. | Page 210 |
| Supine spinal twist | | • Breathe deeply, allowing gravity to guide you into the pose. | Page 178 |
| Final relaxation | | • Let go of any remaining tension.<br>• Stay for as long as time allows. | Page 228 |

# Flex and Flow

Flex and Flow is a one-hour, intermediate-level workout that fuses strength training with total body stretching. The *flex* refers to isometric holds in poses aimed at strengthening and toning your major muscle groups. The *flow* refers to a smooth and fluid series of poses that acts to counterbalance the extensive muscle contracting. This workout alternates flex with flow, simultaneously providing your body with challenge and release.

| MOUNTAIN I: Warm-up | | |
|---|---|---|
| **Standard lying-down warm-up** | | |
| Powerful spinal balance flow | After flowing spinal balance, hold one side for 5 breaths and then flow elbow to opposite knee 3-5 times; change sides. | |
| **VALLEY I: Sun salutations** | | |
| Sun salutations | **Repeat 2-4 times.** | |
| 1. Mountain pose | | • Stand with feet hip-width apart.<br>• Establish a strong base. |
| | | Page 72 |
| 2. Standing forward fold | | • Swan dive into the pose.<br>• Place hands firmly on floor. |
| | | Page 120 |
| 3. Crescent lunge or kneeling lunge | *or* | • Reach back with one foot, maintaining alignment with hip. |
| | | Page 186 |
| 4. Downward-facing dog or child's pose | *or* | • Press back, hinging from the hips. |
| | | Pages 122 and 184 |
| 5. Plank or kneeling plank | *or* | • Draw forward with a neutral spine. |
| | | Page 42 |
| 6. Crocodile or kneeling crocodile | *or* | • Lower upper body while lifting abdominals. |
| | | Page 44 |

> continued

**Flex and Flow** > *continued*

| VALLEY I: Sun salutations | | | |
|---|---|---|---|
| 7. Upward-facing dog or cobra | *or* | • Lift and open the heart.<br>• Lengthen out of lower back. | Pages 48 and 46 |
| 8. Downward-facing dog or child's pose | *or* | • Press back, hinging from the hips. | Pages 122 and 184 |
| 9. Kneeling lunge or crescent lunge | *or* | • Step forward, stacking knee over ankle. | Page 186 |
| 10. Standing forward fold | | • Engage core.<br>• Use reverse swan dive to return to mountain pose. | Page 120 |
| 11. Mountain pose | | • Check in with your body and breath. | Page 72 |
| 12. Chair | | • Relax shoulders back and down.<br>• Keep elbows soft.<br>• Sit back, shifting weight to heels. | Page 94 |
| MOUNTAIN II: Work | | | |
| **Hold poses for 3-5 breaths unless otherwise noted.** | | | |
| **Down dog leg lifts** | | • In downward-facing dog, alternate lifting one leg at a time straight up and back.<br>• Hold each side for 3-5 breaths, then flow from side to side 5 times with your breath. | Page 122 |

| MOUNTAIN II: Work | | | |
|---|---|---|---|
| One-arm down dog | | • In downward-facing dog, place one hand behind your back.<br>• Repeat on both sides. | Page 122 |
| Child's pose | | • Sink hips toward heels. | Page 184 |
| Camel | | • Lift chest and lengthen out of lower back.<br>• Practice expanding breath. | Page 148 |
| Plank push-up series | **First time through the series, hold each pose for 3 breaths. Switch sides. Then, alternate sides 3 times, flowing one breath per movement. Eliminate the one-legged options as desired.** | | |
| 1. Three-legged downward-facing dog | | • From downward-facing dog, lift one leg high to the sky. | Page 122 |
| 2. Upward-facing dog | | • From one-legged plank, place just the tops of both feet on the mat and draw your chest forward. | Page 48 |
| 3. Plank push-up | | • From upward-facing dog, return to plank and lower to crocodile for a "push-up." | Page 42 |
| 4. Downward-facing dog | | • From crocodile, press back to plank and return to downward-facing dog. | Page 122 |
| Crescent lunge | | • Repeat on both sides. | Page 186 |
| Twisting lunge | | • Follow your breath into the rotation.<br>• Let go of judgment. | Page 162 |
| Downward-facing dog | | • Spread the fingers wide.<br>• Lengthen spine.<br>• Bend knees as necessary to lessen intensity. | Page 122 |

> continued

| MOUNTAIN II: Work | | | |
|---|---|---|---|
| Sunflowers | | • Repeat 5 times. | Page 76 |
| Sun pose | | • Practice three-part breath. | Page 78 |
| Chair | | • Relax the shoulders back and down.<br>• Keep the elbows soft.<br>• Sit back, shifting weight to heels. | Page 94 |
| Twisting chair | | • Hold pose for 3-5 breaths on each side.<br>• Alternate sides flowing with the breath 5 times. | Page 166 |
| Warrior II flow | | • Hold warrior II for 3-5 breaths. Then, bend and straighten the forward leg.<br>• Repeat 5 times.<br>• Switch sides. | Page 84 |
| Standing straddle splits | | • For an optional chest expansion, interlace your fingers behind your back and straighten your arms, lifting your knuckles toward the sky. | Page 136 |
| Side angle flow series | **Turn toward back foot and repeat series on other side. Upon completion, turn again to face front of mat.** | | |
| 1. Side angle | | • Sink through hips.<br>• Avoid sinking into bottom hand or shoulder. | Page 90 |
| 2. Side angle arm circles | | • Circle top arm by reaching forward, down and around, 5 times with the breath. | Page 90 |

| MOUNTAIN II: Work | | | |
|---|---|---|---|
| Side angle flow series | **Turn toward back foot and repeat series on other side. Upon completion, turn again to face front of mat.** | | |
| 3. Triangle | | • Maintain neutral spine. | Page 88 |
| 4. Pyramid | | • For an optional chest expansion, interlace your fingers behind your back and straighten your arms, lifting your knuckles toward the sky. | Page 128 |
| 5. Twisting triangle | | • Rotate without rounding your back.<br>• Let go of expectations.<br>• Stay in the present moment. | Page 164 |
| 6. Pyramid | | • Keep hips square with front of mat.<br>• Practice sinking breath to stretch entire back of body. | Page 128 |
| 7. Balancing half moon | | • From pyramid, shift weight to front foot and bring opposite hand to hip or lift to sky.<br>• Come to standing forward fold, and repeat other side. | Page 102 |
| Standing forward fold | | • Engage your core.<br>• Use reverse swan dive to return to mountain pose. | Page 120 |
| Downward-facing dog | | • Pedal feet 10 times. | Page 122 |
| Flow series | **First time through, hold each pose for 3-5 breaths. Then, as usual, flow with the breath. Perform Modified Flow Series instead, if necessary. Repeat 3 times.** | | |
| 1. Downward-facing dog | | • Spread fingers wide.<br>• Lengthen spine.<br>• Bend knees as necessary to lessen intensity. | Page 122 |

> continued

| | MOUNTAIN II: Work | | |
|---|---|---|---|
| **Flow series** | First time through, hold each pose for 3-5 breaths. Then, as usual, flow with the breath.<br>Perform Modified Flow Series instead, if necessary.<br>Repeat 3 times. | | |
| *2. Plank* | | • Draw forward with a neutral spine. | Page 42 |
| *3. Crocodile* | | • Lower upper body while lifting abdominals. | Page 44 |
| *4. Upward-facing dog* | | • Lift and open the heart.<br>• Lengthen out of lower back. | Page 48 |
| *5. Downward-facing dog* | | • Spread fingers wide.<br>• Lengthen spine.<br>• Bend knees as necessary to lessen intensity. | Page 122 |
| **Standing backbend** | | • Establish a strong base.<br>• Lift out of lower back. | Page 144 |
| **Standing chest expansion with forward fold** | | • For lower back discomfort or injury, remain standing upright. | Page 130 |
| VALLEY II: Upright Standing Balance | | | |
| **Dancer** | | • Hold for 5-10 breaths.<br>• Switch sides. | Page 110 |
| **Standing spinal twist** | | • Hold for 5-10 breaths.<br>• Switch sides. | Page 170 |
| MOUNTAIN III: Cool-Down | | | |
| **Hold poses for 5-10 breaths unless otherwise noted.** | | | |
| **Locust** | | • Option to use Superman. | Page 150 |

| MOUNTAIN III: Cool-Down | | | |
|---|---|---|---|
| Bow | | • Watch for signs of struggle.<br>• Create tension without stress. | Page 152 |
| Butterfly boat | | • Hold butterfly for 5 breaths and then inhale to boat (see next pose) and flow between boat and butterfly 2-5 times.<br>• After flowing, hold boat for 5 breaths (option to come into wide toe boat) holding for 5-10 breaths.<br>• End in butterfly, and hold 10 breaths. | Page 200 |
| Boat flow | | • In boat, lean back creating more space between chest and thighs. Exhale back to boat, inhale, open. Move arms as if rowing a boat.<br>• Repeat 5 to 10 times | Page 60 |
| Big-toe wide boat | | • Hold for 5-10 breaths. | Page 62 |
| Butterfly | | • Soften toward floor.<br>• Avoid pulling feet.<br>• Practice sinking breath. | Page 200 |
| Turkish twist | | • Inhale and lengthen.<br>• Exhale and rotate. | Page 176 |
| Dead bug | | • Keep tailbone on floor. | Page 210 |
| Bridge | | • Inhale as you lift into bridge; exhale as you lower your back to the mat.<br>• Repeat 3-5 times. | Page 154 |
| Ab work | | • Bring opposite shoulder, not elbow, to opposite knee. | Page 56 |

> continued

| MOUNTAIN III:  Cool-Down | | | |
|---|---|---|---|
| Bridge | | • Inhale as you lift into bridge, exhale as you lower your back to the mat.<br>• Repeat 3-5 times. | Page 154 |
| Upside-down pigeon | | • Breathe deeply to release tension. | Page 204 |
| Butterfly | | • Soften toward floor.<br>• Avoid pulling feet.<br>• Practice sinking breath. | Page 200 |
| Shoulderstand and plow or legs up the wall | *and*<br><br>*or* | • Practice inversions for greater mental and physical wellbeing.<br>• Keep head in line with spine.<br>• Hold for 5-10 breaths. | Pages 216, 218, and 214 |
| Fish | | • Follows inversions as a counterpose to open throat and chest. | Page 220 |
| Supine spinal twist | | • Breathe deeply, allowing gravity to guide you into the pose. | Page 178 |
| Knees to chest | | • Hold hamstrings and relax to release back. | Page 208 |
| Final relaxation | | • Let go of any remaining tension.<br>• Stay for as long as time allows. | Page 228 |

# YogaCore

YogaCore is a 60- to 75-minute hybrid yoga–fitness workout for intermediate and experienced practitioners. YogaCore targets the midsection and additional muscle groups surrounding and assisting the midsection, including the low back. This workout incorporates more repetition for muscular endurance and involves holding poses for increased strength.

| MOUNTAIN I: Warm-up | | | |
|---|---|---|---|
| Standard Lying-down warm-up | | | |
| VALLEY I: Sun salutations | | | |
| **Sun salutations** | **Repeat 2-4 times.** | | |
| 1. Mountain pose | | • Stand with feet hip-width apart.<br>• Establish a strong base. | Page 72 |
| 2. Standing forward fold | | • Swan dive into the pose.<br>• Place hands firmly on floor. | Page 120 |
| 3. Crescent lunge or kneeling lunge | or | • Reach back with one foot, maintaining alignment with hip. | Page 186 |
| 4. Downward-facing dog or child's pose | or | • Press back, hinging from the hips. | Pages 122 and 184 |
| 5. Plank or kneeling plank | or | • Draw forward with a neutral spine. | Page 42 |
| 6. Crocodile or kneeling crocodile | or | • Lower upper body while lifting abdominals. | Page 44 |
| 7. Upward-facing dog or cobra | or | • Lift and open the heart.<br>• Lengthen out of lower back. | Page 48 and 46 |

> continued

| VALLEY I:  Sun salutations | | | |
|---|---|---|---|
| 8. Downward-facing dog or child's pose | | • Press back, hinging from the hips. | Pages 122 and 184 |
| 9. Crescent lunge or kneeling lunge | | • Step forward, stacking knee over ankle. | Page 186 |
| 10. Standing forward fold | | • Engage core.<br>• Use reverse swan dive to return to mountain. | Page 120 |
| 11. Mountain pose | | • Check in with your body and breath. | Page 72 |
| 12. Chair | | • Relax shoulders back and down.<br>• Keep elbows soft.<br>• Sit back, shifting weight to heels. | Page 94 |
| MOUNTAIN II:  Work | | | |
| **Hold poses for 3-5 breaths unless otherwise noted.** | | | |
| Sun squats | | • From sun pose, inhale while straightening both legs and bring arms overhead; exhale, returning to sun pose.<br>• Repeat 5-10 times. | Page 78 |
| Prayer squat | | • From sun pose lower the hips to knee level or below narrowing width of stance as necessary to keep knees stacked over heels.<br>• Bring hands together at center of chest and hold for 5-10 breaths. | Page 96 |

| MOUNTAIN II: Work | | | |
|---|---|---|---|
| Mountain pose | | • Check in with your body and breath. | Page 72 |
| Standing forward fold | | • Engage core.<br>• Use reverse swan dive to return to mountain pose. | Page 120 |
| Plank | | • From standing forward fold, step, hop, or float back into plank. | Page 42 |
| Side plank lifts | | • From kneeling side plank, lift and lower the extended leg, keeping your toes flexed.<br>• Repeat 5-10 times on each side. | Page 54 |
| Downward-facing dog leg lifts | | • From downward-facing dog, lift one leg at a time straight up and back.<br>• Repeat 5 times on each side. | Page 122 |
| Repeater crescent lunges | | • From crescent lunge, repeatedly pull knee up to chest and return to starting position.<br>• Repeat 5-10 times on each side. | Page 186 |
| Twisting lunge | | • Follow your breath into the rotation.<br>• Let go of judgment. | Page 162 |
| Plank with leg lifts | | • In plank or kneeling plank, lift one leg at a time away from the floor, maintaining a strong core center.<br>• Hold for 5 breaths on each side. | Page 42 |

> continued

| MOUNTAIN II: Work | | | |
|---|---|---|---|
| Full or half side plank | | • Stack wrists and shoulders.<br>• For shoulder injuries or discomfort, place knee on floor below hip. | Page 54 |
| Standing forward fold | | • Engage core.<br>• Use reverse swan dive to return to mountain. | Page 120 |
| Mountain pose | | • Check in with your body and breath. | Page 72 |
| Triangle | | • Maintain neutral spine.<br>• After holding for 5 breaths, bend the forward knee and bring hands to floor inside ankle.<br>• Walk around to standing straddle splits. | Page 88 |
| Standing straddle splits | | • Gently contract your thighs.<br>• Place feet flat on floor with feet parallel to each other.<br>• Lift shoulders away from ears.<br>• Hold for 3-5 breaths. | Page 136 |
| Triangle | | • Walk to opposite foot and set up warrior feet and lift into triangle pose as you straighten legs.<br>• Maintain neutral spine holding for 3-5 breaths.<br>• Return to standing straddle splits. | Page 88 |
| Standing straddle splits | | • Gently contract your thighs.<br>• Place feet flat on floor.<br>• Lift shoulders away from ears. | Page 136 |

| MOUNTAIN II: Work | | | |
|---|---|---|---|
| Prayer squats from standing straddle splits | | • From standing straddle splits bend knees as you walk feet in so heels stack under knees.<br>• Inhale lifting chest and bringing hands together at heart center.<br>• Hug the triceps with the thighs for more dynamic tension, holding for 5 breaths. | Page 96 |
| Standing backbend | | • From prayer squat, stand up and return to mountain pose.<br>• Establish a strong base and place hands on back of hips.<br>• Lift out of low back. | Page 144 |
| VALLEY II: Upright standing balance | | | |
| Standing balance pigeon | | • Hold for 5-10 breaths.<br>• Switch sides. | Page 108 |
| Eagle | | • From standing balance pigeon, bring inner thighs together and keep chest lifted.<br>• The arms intertwine: if the right leg is on top, then right arm is under the left arm.<br>• Gently wrap your body in a hug.<br>• Breathe deeply. | Page 106 |
| MOUNTAIN III: Cool-down | | | |
| Hold poses for 5-10 breaths unless otherwise noted. | | | |
| Downward-facing dog | | • Spread fingers wide.<br>• Lengthen spine.<br>• Bend knees as necessary to lessen intensity. | Page 122 |
| Child's pose | | • Sink hips toward heels. | Page 184 |
| Locust | | • Option to use Superman. | Page 150 |

> continued

| MOUNTAIN III: Cool-down | | | |
|---|---|---|---|
| Bow | | • Watch for signs of struggle.<br>• Create tension without stress. | Page 152 |
| Child's pose | | • Sink hips toward heels. | Page 184 |
| Frog | | • Keep core engaged and knees in line with hips. | Page 198 |
| Seated spinal twist | | • Sit tall. Extend right leg straight and bend left knee, planting foot firmly.<br>• Relax shoulders back and down.<br>• Rotate from bottom to top. | Page 172 |
| Sage pose | | • Keeping the left knee bent, reach left hand toward right foot and reach the right arm around the back. If hands meet, then grasp and release head forward, drawing the navel center inward.<br>• Hold for 5-10 breaths and repeat other side, starting with seated spinal twist (above). | Page 196 |
| Seated straddle splits | | • Point knees and toes up.<br>• Practice sinking breath. | Page 140 |
| Revolving knee to head | | • Keep chest lifted and straight leg engaged.<br>• Heart stays open to sky. | Page 194 |
| Knees to chest | | • Hold hamstrings and relax to release back. | Page 208 |
| Ab work | | • Bring opposite shoulder, not elbow, to opposite knee. | Page 56 |
| Bridge | | • Place feet hip-width apart.<br>• Slide shoulders away from ears before lifting. | Page 154 |

| MOUNTAIN III: Cool-down | | |
|---|---|---|
| **Shoulderstand and plow or legs up the wall** | | • Practice inversions for greater mental and physical wellbeing. <br> • Keep head in line with spine. <br> • Hold for 5-10 breaths. <br><br> *and* <br><br> *or* | Pages 216, 218, and 214 |
| **Fish** | | • Follows inversions as a counterpose to open throat and chest. | Page 220 |
| **Final relaxation** | | • Let go of any remaining tension. <br> • Stay for as long as time allows. | Page 228 |

## Power YogaFit

Power YogaFit is a vigorous 75-minute workout for those who are advanced practitioners of YogaFit or who are in very good physical health. Power YogaFit moves faster for more cardiovascular benefits and also yields increased strength, endurance, balance, and flexibility.

| MOUNTAIN I: Warm-up | | |
|---|---|---|
| **Standard standing warm-up** | | |
| **Powerful spinal balance flow** | After flowing spinal balance, hold one side for 5 breaths and then flow elbow to opposite knee 3-5 times; change sides. | |
| VALLEY I: Sun Salutations | | |
| **Sun Salutations** | **Repeat 2-4 times.** | |
| *1. Mountain pose* | | • Stand with feet hip-width apart. <br> • Establish a strong base. | Page 72 |

> *continued*

| VALLEY I: Sun Salutations | | | |
|---|---|---|---|
| 2. Standing forward fold | | • Swan dive into the pose.<br>• Place hands firmly on floor. | Page 120 |
| 3. Crescent lunge or kneeling lunge | or | • Reach back with one foot, maintaining alignment with hip. | Page 44 |
| 4. Downward-facing dog or child's pose | or | • Press back, hinging from the hips. | Pages 122 and 184 |
| 5. Plank or kneeling plank | or | • Draw forward with a neutral spine. | Page 42 |
| 6. Crocodile or kneeling crocodile | or | • Lower upper body while lifting abdominal muscles. | Page 44 |
| 7. Upward-facing dog or cobra | or | • Lift and open the chest.<br>• Lengthen out of lower back. | Pages 48 and 46 |
| 8. Downward-facing dog or child's pose | or | • Press back, hinging from the hips. | Pages122 and 184 |
| 9. Crescent lunge or kneeling lunge | or | • Step forward, stacking knee over ankle. | Page 186 |
| 10. Standing forward fold | | • Engage core.<br>• Use reverse swan dive to return to mountain pose. | Page 120 |

| VALLEY I:  Sun Salutations | | | |
|---|---|---|---|
| 11. Mountain pose | | • Check in with your body and breath. | Page 72 |
| 12. Chair | | • Relax shoulders back and down.<br>• Keep elbows soft.<br>• Sit back, shifting weight to heels. | Page 94 |

| MOUNTAIN II:  Work | | | |
|---|---|---|---|
| **Hold poses for 3-5 breaths unless otherwise noted.** | | | |
| Downward-facing dog | | • Note that the transition into standing forward fold can be made by stepping, hopping, or floating the feet between the hands. | Page 122 |
| Standing forward fold | | • Engage your core.<br>• Use reverse swan dive to return to mountain pose. | Page 120 |
| Mountain pose | | • Check in with your body and breath. | Page 72 |

| Twisting lunge flow series | **Repeat on both sides.** | | |
|---|---|---|---|
| 1. Downward-facing dog | | • Press back, hinging from the hips. | Page 122 |
| 2. Crescent lunge | | • Step forward, stacking knee over ankle. | Page 186 |
| 3. Twisting lunge | | • Follow your breath into the rotation.<br>• Let go of judgment. | Page 162 |

> continued

| MOUNTAIN II: Work | | | |
|---|---|---|---|
| 4. Downward-facing dog | | • Press back, hinging from the hips. | Page 122 |
| **Twisting chair flow series** | **Repeat 2-4 times, alternating sides.** | | |
| 1. Twisting chair | | • Inhale arms overhead; exhale easing into twisting chair. | Page 166 |
| 2. Side crow | | • From twisting chair place hands to one side shoulder width apart.<br>• Contracting strongly through the belly, glide forward as arms bend to 90 degrees.<br>• Hold for 3-5 breaths. | Page 168 |
| 3. Standing forward fold | | • Exhale into forward fold with bent legs. | Page 120 |
| 4. Reverse swan dive | | • Keep knees bent and spine straight. | Page 236 |
| 5. Twisting chair | | • Keep knees together.<br>• Lift heart to lengthen spine before rotating. | Page 166 |
| **Flow series** | **Repeat 5-10 times.** | | |
| 1. Downward-facing dog | | • Press back, hinging from the hips. | Page 122 |
| 2. Plank | | • Draw forward with a neutral spine. | Page 42 |
| 3. Crocodile | | • Lower upper body while lifting abdominals. | Page 44 |

## MOUNTAIN II: Work

| Flow series | Repeat 5-10 times. | | |
|---|---|---|---|
| 4. Upward-facing dog | | • Lift and open the heart.<br>• Lengthen out of lower back. | Page 48 |
| 5. Downward-facing dog | | • Press back, hinging from the hips. | Page 122 |
| **Plank** | | • Draw forward with a neutral spine. | Page 42 |
| **Downward-facing dog** | | • Spread fingers wide.<br>• Lengthen spine.<br>• Bend knees as necessary to lessen intensity. | Page 122 |
| **Side angle flow series** | **Repeat on each side.** | | |
| 1. Warrior I | | • Press back foot flat to floor.<br>• Square shoulders with front of mat.<br>• Point tailbone towards floor. | Page 82 |
| 2. Warrior II | | • Face long edge of mat.<br>• Stack forward knee over ankle. | Page 84 |
| 3. Reverse warrior | | • Remember to side bend, not back bend. | Page 86 |
| 4. Side angle | | • Sink through hips.<br>• Avoid sinking into bottom hand or shoulder. | Page 90 |
| **Flow series** | **(See Flow Series earlier in this workout)** | • **Repeat 3-5 times.** | |

> continued

| MOUNTAIN II: Work | | | |
|---|---|---|---|
| Downward-facing dog | | • Spread fingers wide.<br>• Lengthen spine.<br>• Bend knees as necessary to lessen intensity. | Page 122 |
| **Prayer twisting flow series** | **Repeat on each side.** | | |
| 1. Crescent lunge | | • For less intensity, place fingers on floor or drop back knee. | Page 186 |
| 2. Prayer twisting lunge | | • Practice dynamic tension and surrender. | Page 162 |
| 3. Standing straddle splits | | • Gently contract your thighs.<br>• Place feet flat on floor.<br>• Lift shoulders away from ears. | Page 136 |
| 4. Crescent lunge | | • For less intensity, place fingers on floor or drop back knee. | Page 186 |
| 5. Downward-facing dog | | • Spread fingers wide.<br>• Lengthen spine.<br>• Bend knees as necessary to lessen intensity. | Page 122 |
| **Standing forward fold** | | • Engage your core.<br>• Use reverse swan dive to return to mountain pose. | Page 120 |
| **Standing backbend** | | • Establish a strong base.<br>• Lift out of low back. | Page 144 |

| MOUNTAIN II: Work | | | |
|---|---|---|---|
| **Standing chest expansion with forward fold** | | • For low-back discomfort or injury, remain standing upright. | Page 130 |
| **Mountain pose** | | • Check in with your body and breath. | Page 72 |
| **Triangle series** | Repeat series on both sides. | | |
| *1. Triangle* | | • Maintain neutral spine. | Page 88 |
| *2. Side angle* | | • Sink through hips.<br>• Avoid sinking into bottom hand or shoulder. | Page 90 |
| *3. Bound side angle* | | • From side angle pose reach bottom hand under thigh and top hand behind back keeping torso stacking over thigh.<br>• Hold for 5-10 breaths<br>• Hands can be clasped or not. | Page 92 |
| *4. Bound triangle* | | • From bound side angle straighten front leg.<br>• Keep chest open. | Page 92 |
| **Standing straddle splits with chest expansion arms** | | • Place hands on hips or interlace fingers together and lift shoulders away from ears.<br>• Gently contract your thighs.<br>• Place feet flat on floor. | Page 136 |

> *continued*

| MOUNTAIN II: Work | | | |
|---|---|---|---|
| **Prayer squat to bird of paradise** | *to* | • From standing straddle splits, bend knees and lift into prayer squat with feet hip-width apart.<br>• Wrap right arm in front of right thigh and around back, clasping left hand from behind and binding the hands together, or use a towel.<br>• Press into the left foot, straightening left leg, and lift right leg and chest toward the sky.<br>• Hold for 3-5 breaths, release into squat, and repeat other side. | Pages 96 and 114 |
| **Standing forward fold** | | • Engage your core.<br>• Use reverse swan dive to return to mountain pose. | Page 120 |
| **Dolphin and plank flow series** | **Repeat series 3-5 times.** | | |
| *1. Plank* | | • Draw forward with a neutral spine. | Page 42 |
| *2. Child's pose* | | • Sink hips toward heels. | Page 184 |
| *3. Dolphin* | | • From child's pose, inhale, bringing chin over thumbs; exhale, pressing back to dolphin. | Page 124 |
| **Downward-facing dog** | | • Spread fingers wide.<br>• Lengthen spine.<br>• Bend knees as necessary to lessen intensity. | Page 122 |
| **Three-legged downward-facing dog** | | • From downward-facing dog, lift one leg high to the sky.<br>• Repeat on each side. | Page 122 |

| MOUNTAIN II: Work | | | |
|---|---|---|---|
| Side plank | | • Stack wrists and shoulders.<br>• For shoulder injuries or discomfort, place knee on floor below hip. | Page 54 |
| Child's pose | | • Sink hips toward heels. | Page 184 |

| VALLEY II: Upright standing balance | | | |
|---|---|---|---|
| **Hold poses for 5-10 breaths unless otherwise noted.** | | | |
| Warrior III | | • Option to transition directly from warrior III to eagle by bringing the elevated leg forward and wrapping it around the standing leg.<br>• Bend the standing leg and engage root lock (chapter 3) for a safer transition. | Page 98 |
| Eagle | | • Gently wrap your body in a hug.<br>• Breathe deeply. | Page 106 |
| Big toe hold | | • Keep both hips on the mat, bending knees as necessary.<br>• Switch sides.<br>• Hold each phase for 5 breaths. | Page 212 |

| MOUNTAIN III: Cool-down | | | |
|---|---|---|---|
| **Hold poses for 5-10 breaths unless otherwise noted.** | | | |
| Seated forward fold | | • Draw forward using your lower abdominals. | Page 138 |
| Tabletop | | • Option to flow from tabletop to boat 3 times. | Page 52 |
| Boat | | • Option to flow from tabletop to boat 3 times. | Page 60 |
| Ab work | | • Bring opposite shoulder, not elbow, to opposite knee. | Page 56 |

> *continued*

| MOUNTAIN III: Cool-down | | | |
|---|---|---|---|
| **Seated spinal twist** | | • Sit tall.<br>• Relax shoulders back and down.<br>• Rotate from bottom to top. | Page 172 |
| **Turkish twist** | | • Inhale and lengthen.<br>• Exhale and rotate. | Page 176 |
| **Elephant** | | • From a seated pose, bend right leg, inserting right arm under right leg.<br>• Hook left ankle on top of right.<br>• Place hands firmly on the ground shoulder-width apart, and contract abdominal muscles strongly as you press hands into the floor and lift buttocks off floor. | Page 66 |
| **Eight-angle pose** | | • From balancing elephant pose, bend the elbows as you squeeze the inner thighs together pressing right heels out to the side extending both legs.<br>• Hold for 3-5 breaths, and repeat other side starting with elephant. | Page 66 |
| **Dead bug** | | • Keep tailbone on floor. | Page 210 |
| **Bridge or wheel** | *or* | • Expect increased energy and alertness.<br>• Practice expanding breath. | Pages 154 and 156 |
| **Big toe hold** | | • This pose combines strength, flexibility, effort, and surrender.<br>• Hold each phase for 5 breaths. | Page 212 |

| MOUNTAIN III: Cool-down | | | |
|---|---|---|---|
| **Knees to chest** | | • Hold hamstrings and relax to release back. | Page 208 |
| **L-shaped forearm balance and L-shaped handstand or legs up the wall** | *and*<br><br>*or* | • L-shaped forearm: start in dolphin pose with heels against the wall. Activate the core as you walk feet up the wall to hip level.<br>• Establish pada bandha and press firmly into the floor with forearms.<br>• L-shaped handstand: Start in downward-facing dog with heels against the wall. Walk feet up the wall to hip level, and press firmly into the wall maintaining pada bandha.<br>• Press firmly through fingers, and maintain shoulders over wrists. | Pages 226, 224, and 214 |
| **Fish** | | • Follows inversions as a counterpose to open throat and chest. | Page 220 |
| **Final relaxation** | | • Let go of any remaining tension.<br>• Stay for as long as time allows. | Page 228 |

## Taking Your Workout to the Next Level

There's always a next step in YogaFit. There's no such thing as mastering a pose, no matter how basic it seems, because every day your body is different, and your circumstances are different, ensuring that you'll always find a new place to go.

However, as you become stronger and more flexible, you might want more from your practice. Whether you stay with the Beginning YogaFit format, or progress to Power Yoga, you can always make any format more challenging through these simple modifications:

- Increase the number of sun salutations in valley I.
- Hold mountain II poses for longer than three to five breaths. As long as you can maintain a steady, deep breath, without experiencing pain, you can stay as long as you like.

- Use the flow series in mountains I and II. Add repetitions of this flow, on or off the knees, wherever you like to create more heat, increase your heart rate, and build strength.

- Hold mountain III poses for longer than 10 breaths. As long as you can maintain a steady, deep breath, without experiencing pain, you can stay as long as you like.

- Move through the poses with only one or two breaths in each pose for a more cardiovascular workout.

# Sport-Specific Poses

YogaFit was created out of a need to bring yoga to the everyday person and the weekend athlete who perhaps would not have ever considered walking into a yoga studio! Times have changed in the 20 years since YogaFit introduced yoga into the gym atmosphere and has served as an introduction of the benefits of yoga for many hundreds of thousands of people. YogaFit is the perfect complement for professional athletes, weekend warriors, and people interested in getting a good, total body–mind workout. Traditional exercise programs often overwork certain muscle groups or build muscle bulk unevenly, and perhaps more importantly, are not focused on the breath. They tend to neglect training participants to breathe efficiently or to improve their mental game. YogaFit can be extremely helpful in counteracting some of the negative effects of these traditional programs and in expanding programs to focus on more than just muscular strength. Many professional athletes have turned to yoga as a tool for abating injury. For example, many teams in the NFL require their players to practice yoga as an adjunct workout. YogaFit trains both the mental and the physical bodies in a way that traditional exercise cannot.

As an athlete, you can and will benefit from a regular YogaFit workout, but you might also want to complement your practice with sport-specific poses for strengthening, stretching, endurance, balance, focus, and relaxation. Use these poses either before or after your regular workout or training, or between weightlifting sets. Sun salutations provide a great dynamic stretch and warm-up before any athletic event. Moving a muscle in its range of motion is more effective as a warm-up than static stretching prior to any athletic event. A YogaFit practice will enhance your efforts in any given sport or just at creating more movement through the years.

As always, before practicing any of the following poses, review part I as well as the corresponding pose pages in part II.

Dynamic warm-up for any sport: Perform two to six times either kneeling or full. If your activity involves twisting, such as tennis or golf, then adding a twisting lunge to the sun salutation will be beneficial.

# Swimming

Swimming and YogaFit have much in common in that both focus on moving and breathing rhythmically. For all levels of swimmers, YogaFit breathing is key—first, learning to unite the breath with movement in the water, and then practicing specific breathing techniques out of the water in order to improve concentration, breath control, and endurance. YogaFit poses can help balance the strength swimmers build in their upper bodies and shoulders with flexibility, for a healthier range of motion. Also, because swimming favors the upper body at the expense of the legs and core muscles, standing poses such as the warrior poses and the chair, along with abdominal work on the floor, can help your body maintain muscular balance.

| STRENGTH FOCUS | | | |
|---|---|---|---|
| Ab work | | • One breath per movement. | Page 56 |
| Locust or Superman | *or* | • Hold for 5-10 breaths. | Page 150 |
| Incline plank | | • Hold for 5-10 breaths. | Page 50 |
| Warrior I | | • Hold for 3-5 breaths. | Page 82 |
| Warrior II | | • Hold for 3-5 breaths. | Page 84 |
| Warrior III | | • Hold for 5-10 breaths. | Page 98 |
| **FLEXIBILITY FOCUS** | | | |
| Standing chest expansion with forward fold | | • Hold for 3-5 breaths. | Page 130 |

> *continued*

| FLEXIBILITY FOCUS | | | |
|---|---|---|---|
| Standing backbend | | • Hold for 5-10 breaths. | Page 144 |
| Kneeling shoulder stretch | | • Hold for 5-10 breaths. | Page 192 |
| Camel | | • Hold for 5-10 breaths. | Page 148 |
| Bow | | • Hold for 5-10 breaths. | Page 152 |
| Sage pose | | • Inhale deeply while holding the pose, and exhale, drawing navel strongly inward with long, slow exhalations.<br>• Hold for 5-10 breaths. | Page 196 |
| Turtle | | • Hold for 5-10 breaths. | Page 202 |
| Half lord of the fishes | | • Hold for 5-10 breaths. | Page 174 |
| Bridge | | • Hold for 5-10 breaths. | Page 154 |
| Fish | | • Hold for 5-10 breaths. | Page 220 |

Additional practice
• Practice three-part breath and other breathing techniques for more efficient, focused, and intense workouts (see chapter 3).
• Improve performance through meditation and visualization.
• Perform any standing balance poses (see chapter 6).

# Running

Because of the repetitive motion of the legs, running creates tightness in the hip flexors, hamstrings, and quads, often leading to low-back pain. Running also fails to strengthen the upper body or the abdominal muscles. The YogaFit poses here serve as counterposes to offset runners' lower-body strength and to provide supplemental work to increase total body strength, endurance, and flexibility. After a run is a great time to add in some fun arm balances and then move to the floor for increasing upper-body and core strength. Many runners find that yoga keeps them running longer and faster, without the nagging injuries.

| STRENGTH FOCUS | | | |
|---|---|---|---|
| Ab work | | • One breath per movement. | Page 56 |
| Modified flow series | **One breath per movement.** **You can perform the Flow Series instead (pages 262-263).** | | |
| 1. Child's pose | | • Sink hips toward heels. | Page 184 |
| 2. Kneeling plank | | • Draw forward with a neutral spine. | Page 42 |
| 3. Kneeling crocodile | | • Lower upper body while lifting abdominals. | Page 44 |
| 4. Cobra | | • Lift and open the heart. <br> • Lengthen out of lower back. | Page 46 |
| Prayer squats | | • Maintain strong base and keeping knees stacking over heels. Lower hips to appropriate level for you. <br> • Hold for 3-5 breaths | Page 96 |

> continued

| STRENGTH FOCUS | | | |
|---|---|---|---|
| Crow | | • From prayer squat, place hands on the floor shoulder width apart. Hugging triceps with inner thighs, glide forward as the elbows bend.<br>• Contract abdominal muscles strongly, and tuck feet up, keeping gaze forward.<br>• Hold for 3-5 breaths. | Page 64 |
| Dancer | | • From mountain pose, hold right ankle with right hand and hinge forward at left hip while left hand reaches skyward.<br>• Keep heart lifted and left foot grounded.<br>• Hold for 3-5 breaths and repeat other side. | Page 110 |
| Standing big toe hold | | • From mountain pose, lift right knee as high as possible so right hand reaches right ankle or foot.<br>• Keeping core strong and spine neutral, extend right leg out to front and then to side.<br>• Can be holding foot or ankle or not bind hands at all.<br>• Hold for 3-5 breaths, and repeat other side. | Page 112 |
| FLEXIBILITY FOCUS | | | |
| Kneeling lunge | | • Hold for 5-10 breaths. | Page 186 |
| Quadriceps stretch | | • Hold for 5-10 breaths. | Page 188 |
| Bow | | • Hold for 5-10 breaths. | Page 152 |

| FLEXIBILITY FOCUS | | | |
|---|---|---|---|
| Incline plank | | • Hold for 5-10 breaths. | Page 50 |
| Seated forward fold | | • Hold for 5-10 breaths. | Page 138 |
| Butterfly | | • Hold for 5-10 breaths. | Page 200 |
| Revolving head to knee | | • Hold for 5-10 breaths. | Page 194 |
| Upside-down pigeon | | • Hold for 5-10 breaths. | Page 204 |

Additional practice
• Practice three-part breath and other breathing techniques for more efficient, focused, and intense workouts (see chapter 3).
• Improve performance through meditation and visualization.
• Perform any standing balance poses, especially tree and dancer (see chapter 6).

# Cycling

Like running, cycling requires repetitive motion that shortens and tightens certain leg muscles while underusing others. Cycling also overstretches and underuses certain muscles in the upper back and abdomen, leading to postural alignment issues and (in some cases) back pain. In YogaFit, cyclists should focus on poses that counteract the seated and forward-reaching position they adopt in cycling; they should also do deep stretches that target their legs and hips. Practiced regularly, these poses help cyclists feel better longer, on and off the bike.

| STRENGTH FOCUS | | | |
|---|---|---|---|
| **Ab work** | | • One breath per movement. | Page 56 |
| **Modified flow series** | One breath per movement.<br>**You can perform Flow Series instead (pages 262-263).** | | |
| 1. *Child's pose* | | • Sink hips toward heels. | Page 184 |
| 2. *Kneeling plank* | | • Draw forward with a neutral spine. | Page 42 |
| 3. *Cobra* | | • Lift and open the heart.<br>• Lengthen out of lower back. | Page 46 |
| 4. *Kneeling crocodile* | | • Lower upper body while lifting abdominal muscles. | Page 44 |
| 5. *Child's pose* | | • Sink hips toward heels. | Page 184 |
| **Standing straddle splits** | | • Gently contract your thighs.<br>• Place feet flat on floor with feet parallel to each other.<br>• Lift shoulders away from ears.<br>• Hold for 3-5 breaths. | Page 136 |
| **Triangle** | | • From standing straddle splits, walk hands around to left side. Point left foot forward, and straighten legs, lifting chest center with spine in neutral. Left hand can be on thigh, knee, or ankle.<br>• Reach both hands out in opposite directions, and ground through the feet.<br>• Maintain neutral spine, and lift through the chest center.<br>• Repeat other side. | Page 88 |

| STRENGTH FOCUS | | | |
|---|---|---|---|
| Pyramid | | • From triangle turn back foot forward and step foot closer to square hips toward top of mat.<br>• Hinge at the front hip, keeping spine in neutral, and support hands on thigh; or move deeper, keeping stretch in the front hamstrings.<br>• Hold for 3-5 breaths. | Page 128 |
| Crow | | • From squat, place hands on the floor shoulder-width apart. Hugging triceps with inner thighs, glide forward as the elbows bend.<br>• Contract abs strongly and tuck feet up, keeping gaze forward.<br>• Hold for 3-5 breaths. | Page 64 |
| FLEXIBILITY FOCUS | | | |
| Dancer | | • From mountain pose, hold right ankle with right hand and hinge forward at left hip while left hand reaches skyward.<br>• Keep heart lifted and left foot grounded.<br>• Hold for 3-5 breaths and repeat other side. | Page 110 |
| Kneeling lunge | | • Hold for 5-10 breaths. | Page 186 |
| Frog | | • Hold for 5-10 breaths. | Page 198 |
| Bow | | • Hold for 5-10 breaths. | Page 152 |
| Upside-down pigeon | | • Hold for 5-10 breaths. | Page 204 |

> continued

**Cycling** > *continued*

| FLEXIBILITY FOCUS | | | |
|---|---|---|---|
| Supine half lotus | | • Lying on your back, let left ankle rest on right thigh with knee bent. Support left knee as needed to keep hips grounded and level.<br>• Hold 5-10 breaths, and repeat other side. | Page 206 |
| Bridge | | • Hold for 5-10 breaths. | Page 154 |

Additional practice
• Practice three-part breath and other breathing techniques for more efficient, focused, and intense workouts (see chapter 3).
• Improve performance through meditation and visualization.
• Perform shoulder rolls.
• Perform any standing balance poses, especially tree and dancer (see chapter 6).

## Golf

A common complaint among golfers is low-back pain. Golfers lean forward as they stand, which causes back strain, and they aggravate this strain by swinging in the same direction more than 100 times a round. Even just a few YogaFit poses to strengthen the back and rotate the spine in both directions can go a long way toward increasing power and decreasing tension for golfers. Improved concentration and relaxation through meditation and visualization can give a golfer the edge necessary to master what is largely a mental game. The physical benefits of the increased flexibility cannot be ignored. For example, a YogaFit Level 1 trainee in Massachusetts was a 30-something high school football coach who had been assigned to teach yoga to the players in fall and needed to learn. He tolerated the weekend and even had a little fun. Monday afternoon after his golf game, he called to report that his golf drive was 100 yards longer and wanted to know if that was the YogaFit. Before you play golf, warm up with four to six modified sun salutations, adding a kneeling twisting lunge.

| STRENGTH FOCUS | | | |
|---|---|---|---|
| Ab work | | • One breath per movement. | Page 56 |

| STRENGTH FOCUS | | | |
|---|---|---|---|
| **Modified flow series** | One breath per movement. You can perform Flow Series instead (pages 262-263). | | |
| *1. Child's pose* | | • Sink hips toward heels. | Page 184 |
| *2. Kneeling plank* | | • Draw forward with a neutral spine. | Page 42 |
| *3. Cobra* | | • Lift and open the heart. <br> • Lengthen out of lower back. | Page 46 |
| *4. Kneeling crocodile* | | • Lower upper body while lifting abdominals. | Page 44 |
| *5. Child's pose* | | • Sink hips toward heels. | Page 184 |
| *6. Dancer* | | • From mountain pose, hold right ankle with right hand and hinge forward at left hip while left hand reaches skyward. <br> • Keep heart lifted and left foot grounded. <br> • Hold for 3-5 breaths, and repeat other side. | Page 110 |
| *7. Standing spinal twist* | | • From mountain pose lift right leg with knee bent. <br> • With hands at chest center twist toward the right keeping hips square. <br> • Keep hands at chest, or hold right knee with left hand. <br> • Option to bind right hand to left toe and reach left hand back deepening the sensation of the twist. | Page 170 |
| **Bridge** | | • Hold for 5-10 breaths. | Page 154 |

> continued

| FLEXIBILITY FOCUS | | | |
|---|---|---|---|
| Locust | | • Hold for 5-10 breaths. | Page 150 |
| Kneeling lunge | | • Hold for 5-10 breaths. | Page 186 |
| Kneeling shoulder stretch | | • Hold for 5-10 breaths each side. | Page 192 |
| Camel | | • From kneeling, place hands on back of hip bones.<br>• Drop shoulder blades down and squeeze closer as you lift the heart.<br>• Keep head in line with spine.<br>• Hold for 5-10 breaths. | Page 148 |
| Seated spinal twist | | • Hold for 5-10 breaths. | Page 172 |
| Sage pose | | • From a seated pose bend the left knee, reach left hand toward right foot, and reach the right arm around the back. If hands meet, then grasp and release head forward, drawing the navel center inward.<br>• Hold for 5-10 breaths, and repeat other side. | Page 196 |
| Upside-down pigeon | | • Hold for 5-10 breaths. | Page 204 |

Additional practice
• Practice relaxation breath for focus and concentration (see chapter 3).
• Improve mental game through meditation and visualization.
• Perform standing lateral flexion (see chapter 6).
• Perform any twists (see chapter 8).
• Perform any standing balance poses (see chapter 6).
• Perform shoulder rolls and stretches.

# Tennis

Tennis players favor one side of the body and place huge demands on the dominant shoulder, shortening their range of motion and creating other imbalances in the upper body and spine that can lead to pain and injury. Tennis also causes tightness in the hips and hamstrings, which can result in back pain. YogaFit poses help create length in both sides of the torso, rotate the spine in both directions for balance, and promote both strength and flexibility in and around the shoulders, which is critical for stability and a powerful serve. The dynamic nature of a YogaFit practice, especially flowing in the warrior poses, is beneficial to tennis players; they mimic the movements on the court. One recreational tennis player confided in me that her players began to call her "Gumby" after a year of her YogaFit practice. She was able to increase her net presence and poaching ability because of the strength increases she gained in her practice.

| STRENGTH FOCUS | | | |
|---|---|---|---|
| Ab work | | • One breath per movement. | Page 56 |
| Modified flow series | **One breath per movement.** **You can perform Flow Series instead (pages 262-263).** | | |
| 1. Child's pose | | • Sink hips toward heels. | Page 184 |
| 2. Kneeling plank | | • Draw forward with a neutral spine. | Page 42 |
| 3. Cobra | | • Lift and open the heart.<br>• Lengthen out of lower back. | Page 46 |
| 4. Kneeling crocodile | | • Lower upper body while lifting abdominals. | Page 44 |
| 5. Child's pose | | • Sink hips toward heels. | Page 184 |
| Downward-facing dog | | • Hold for 3-5 breaths. | Page 122 |

> continued

| STRENGTH FOCUS | | | |
|---|---|---|---|
| **Warrior II** | | • Hold for 3-5 breaths. | Page 84 |
| **Side angle** | | • Hold for 3-5 breaths. | Page 90 |
| **Reverse warrior** | | • Hold for 3-5 breaths. | Page 86 |
| **Twisting lunge** | | • Hold for 3-5 breaths. | Page 162 |
| **Side crow** | | • From twisting lunge, place hands on floor on outside of bent knee, shoulder-with apart.<br>• Contracting strongly through the belly, glide forward as arms bend to 90 degrees.<br>• Hold for 3-5 breaths. | Page 168 |
| FLEXIBILITY FOCUS | | | |
| **Standing balance pigeon** | | • Hold for 3-5 breaths. | Page 108 |
| **Dancer** | | • Hold for 3-5 breaths. | Page 110 |

| FLEXIBILITY FOCUS | | | |
|---|---|---|---|
| Standing chest expansion with forward fold | | • Hold for 3-5 breaths. | Page 130 |
| Kneeling shoulder stretch | | • Hold for 5-10 breaths. | Page 192 |
| Camel | | • Hold for 5-10 breaths. | Page 148 |
| Frog | | • Hold for 5-10 breaths. | Page 198 |
| Bridge | | • Hold for 5-10 breaths | Page 154 |
| Shoulderstand | | • Hold for 5-10 breaths. | Page 216 |
| Fish | | • Option to put block under head for more support.<br>• Hold for 5-10 breaths. | Page 220 |
| Supine spinal twist | | • Hold for 5-10 breaths. | Page 178 |

Additional practice
• Practice relaxation breath for focus and concentration (see chapter 3).
• Improve mental game through meditation and visualization.
• Perform standing lateral flexion (see chapter 6).
• Perform any twists (see chapter 8).
• Perform any standing balance poses (see chapter 6).
• Perform shoulder rolls and stretches.

## Baseball and Softball

Baseball and softball players favor one side of the body and tend to shorten their range of motion, creating imbalances that can lead to pain and injury. Softball and baseball cause tightness in the hips, quadriceps, and hamstrings, so players might develop back pain. In addition, these games require a flexible torso, which can be developed and maintained through twists. Because these sports strongly favor a dominant side, YogaFit poses are necessary to prevent dramatic imbalances and to increase strength on the weaker side. Focusing on balancing right and left increases the strength of the whole body, making for better performance and less pain.

| STRENGTH FOCUS | | | |
|---|---|---|---|
| Ab work | | • One breath per movement. | Page 56 |
| Modified flow series | One breath per movement. You can perform Flow Series instead (pages 262-263). | | |
| 1. Child's pose | | • Sink hips toward heels. | Page 184 |
| 2. Kneeling plank | | • Draw forward with a neutral spine. | Page 42 |
| 3. Cobra | | • Lift and open the heart.<br>• Lengthen out of lower back. | Page 46 |
| 4. Kneeling crocodile | | • Lower upper body while lifting abdominals. | Page 44 |
| 5. Child's pose | | • Sink hips toward heels. | Page 184 |
| FLEXIBILITY FOCUS | | | |
| Standing chest expansion with forward fold | | • Hold for 3-5 breaths. | Page 130 |

| | | | |
|---|---|---|---|
| **Dancer** | | • Keep lifting through the chest.<br>• Hold for 3-5 breaths. | Page 110 |
| **Eagle** | | • Relax shoulders down and breathe into the back to broaden.<br>• Hold for 3-5 breaths. | Page 106 |
| **Kneeling shoulder stretch** | | • Hold for 5-10 breaths. | Page 192 |
| **Frog** | | • Hold for 5-10 breaths. | Page 198 |
| **Sage pose** | | • Hold for 5-10 breaths. | Page 196 |
| **Seated spinal twist** | | • Inhale while lengthening the spine, and exhale while rotating the spine.<br>• Hold for 5-10 breaths each side. | Page 172 |
| **Big toe hold** | | • Hold for 5 breaths with upper body lifted toward leg for more core activation.<br>• Hold for 5 breaths with leg out to side for opening the hips. | Page 212 |
| **Upside-down pigeon** | | • Hold for 5-10 breaths. | Page 204 |
| **Bow** | | • Hold for 5-10 breaths. | Page 152 |
| **Bridge** | | • Hold for 5-10 breaths. | Page 154 |

*> continued*

**Baseball and Softball**  > *continued*

| FLEXIBILITY FOCUS | | | |
|---|---|---|---|
| **Dead bug** | | • Hold for 5-10 breaths. | Page 210 |

Additional practice
• Practice relaxation breath for focus and concentration (see chapter 3).
• Improve mental game through meditation and visualization.
• Perform standing lateral flexion (see chapter 6).
• Perform any twists (see chapter 8).
• Perform any standing balance poses, especially eagle (see chapter 6).
• Perform shoulder rolls and stretches.

## Volleyball and Basketball

Volleyball and basketball are popular recreational sports, but over time they tend to demand more than the body can give, leading to shoulder and knee injuries. Whether players play for fun or competitively, they should balance the demands of these sports with yoga poses that stretch and strengthen the shoulders and back, stabilize their knees, and increase their core strength for jumps and low-back support. Athletes in these sports should also increase their cardiovascular endurance through breathing practices that strengthen the diaphragm.

| STRENGTH FOCUS | | | |
|---|---|---|---|
| **Ab Work** | | • One breath per movement. | Page 56 |
| **Modified flow series** | **One breath per movement.** **You can perform flow series instead (pages 262-263).** | | |
| *1. Standing big toe hold* | | • Ground through the standing leg<br>• Switch sides.<br>• Hold each side for 3-5 breaths. | Page 112 |
| *2. Child's pose* | | • Sink hips toward heels. | Page 184 |

| STRENGTH FOCUS | | | |
|---|---|---|---|
| **Modified flow series** | **One breath per movement.**<br>**You can perform flow series instead (pages 262-263).** | | |
| *3. Kneeling plank* | | • Draw forward with a neutral spine. | Page 42 |
| *4. Cobra* | | • Lift and open the heart.<br>• Lengthen out of lower back. | Page 46 |
| *5. Kneeling crocodile* | | • Lower upper body while lifting abdominals muscles. | Page 44 |
| *6. Child's pose* | | • Sink hips toward heels. | Page 184 |
| **Warrior I** | | • Hold for 3-5 breaths. | Page 82 |
| FLEXIBILITY FOCUS | | | |
| **Kneeling shoulder stretch** | | • Hold for 5-10 breaths. | Page 192 |
| **Camel** | | • Hold for 5-10 breaths. | Page 148 |
| **Frog** | | • Hold for 5-10 breaths. | Page 198 |
| **Locust** | | • Inhale into locust and hold for 5-10 breaths, focusing on slow exhalations. | Page 150 |
| **Bow** | | • Hold for 5-10 breaths. | Page 152 |

> continued

**Volleyball and Basketball**  > *continued*

| FLEXIBILITY FOCUS | | | |
|---|---|---|---|
| Seated forward fold | | • Hold for 5-10 breaths. | Page 120 |
| Incline plank | | • Hold for 5-10 breaths. | Page 50 |
| Bridge | | • Hold for 5-10 breaths. | Page 154 |
| Upside-down pigeon | | • Hold for 5-10 breaths. | Page 204 |

Additional practice
• Practice three-part breath and other breathing techniques for more efficient, focused, and intense workouts (see chapter 3).
• Improve mental game through meditation and visualization.
• Perform standing lateral flexion (see chapter 6).
• Perform any twists (see chapter 8).
• Perform any standing balance poses, especially eagle (see chapter 6).
• Perform shoulder rolls and stretches.

# Skiing and Snowboarding

Balance is a primary focus for skiers and snowboarders, as is stretching the lower body, including the hips, quadriceps, and hamstrings. As with all sports that overwork these muscles, chronic muscular tension and back pain might be an issue. Athletes in these sports should focus on core strength in order to assist their balance on the slopes and to support their backs. They should also perform deep and relaxing stretches to offset time spent crouched and controlled.

| STRENGTH FOCUS | | | |
|---|---|---|---|
| **Ab work** | | • One breath per movement. | Page 56 |
| **Modified flow series** | **One breath per movement. You can perform Flow Series instead (pages 262-263).** | | |
| 1. *Child's pose* | | • Sink hips toward heels. | Page 184 |
| 2. *Kneeling plank* | | • Draw forward with a neutral spine. | Page 42 |
| 3. *Cobra* | | • Lift and open the heart.<br>• Lengthen out of lower back. | Page 46 |
| 4. *Kneeling crocodile* | | • Lower upper body while lifting abdominals muscles. | Page 44 |
| 5. *Child's pose* | | • Sink hips toward heels. | Page 184 |
| **Chair** | | • Hold for 3-5 breaths. | Page 94 |
| **Twisting chair** | | • Hold for 3-5 breaths. | Page 166 |

> *continued*

| STRENGTH FOCUS | | | |
|---|---|---|---|
| Crow | | • Hold for 3-5 breaths. | Page 64 |
| Downward-facing dog | | • Hold for 3-5 breaths. | Page 122 |
| L-shaped handstand | | • Hold for 3-5 breaths. | Page 224 |
| L-shaped forearm balance | | • Hold for 3-5 breaths. | Page 226 |

| FLEXIBILITY FOCUS | | | |
|---|---|---|---|
| Standing chest expansion with forward fold | | • Hold for 3-5 breaths. | Page 130 |
| Camel | | • Hold for 5-10 breaths. | Page 148 |
| Warrior III | | • Hold for 3-5 breaths. | Page 98 |

| FLEXIBILITY FOCUS | | | |
|---|---|---|---|
| Dancer | | • Hold for 3-5 breaths. | Page 110 |
| Eagle | | • Hold for 3-5 breaths. | Page 106 |
| Kneeling lunge | | • Hold for 5-10 breaths. | Page 186 |
| Quadriceps stretch | | • Hold for 5-10 breaths. | Page 188 |
| Frog | | • Hold for 5-10 breaths. | Page 198 |
| Turtle | | • Hold for 5-10 breaths. | Page 202 |
| Upside-down pigeon | | • Hold for 5-10 breaths. | Page 204 |
| Bridge | | • Hold for 5-10 breaths. | Page 154 |

Additional practice
• Practice three-part breath and other breathing techniques for more efficient, focused, and intense workouts (see chapter 3).
• Improve mental game through meditation and visualization.
• Perform any twists (see chapter 8).
• Perform any standing balance poses, especially balancing half moon, tree, and warrior III (see chapter 6).
• Perform shoulder rolls and stretches.

## Weightlifting

Weightlifting, an integral part of most sports and fitness programs, is best complemented by poses that increase flexibility. Incorporating YogaFit poses and sequences into a weightlifting training program promotes healthy joints and strong, flexible muscles and tendons, benefiting athletes and fitness enthusiasts alike.

| BETWEEN SETS | | | |
|---|---|---|---|
| Standing chest expansion with forward fold | | • Hold for 3-5 breaths. | Page 130 |
| Downward-facing dog | | • Hold for 3-5 breaths. | Page 122 |
| Bow | | • Hold for 5-10 breaths. | Page 152 |
| **FLEXIBILITY FOCUS** | | | |
| Pyramid | | • Hold for 3-5 breaths. | Page 128 |
| Standing backbend | | • Hold for 3-5 breaths. | Page 144 |
| Camel | | • Hold for 5-10 breaths. | Page 148 |
| Kneeling shoulder stretch | | • Hold for 5-10 breaths. | Page 192 |

# Kickboxing and Boxing

Boxing and kickboxing create tightness in the shoulders and hips and are potentially hard on the knees and back. Because these sports tend to be quite aerobic, athletes should practice deep breathing for maximum efficiency and focus. They can balance the explosive movements of their sports with YogaFit poses that help keep the joints stable and mobile. Flexibility and balance are critical for strength and agility, so boxers and kickboxers should perform deep stretches and standing balance poses regularly.

| STRENGTH FOCUS | | | |
|---|---|---|---|
| Ab work | | • One breath per movement. | Page 56 |
| Downward-facing dog | | • Hold for 3-5 breaths. | Page 122 |
| Spinal balance | | • Hold for 3-5 breaths. | Page 58 |
| **FLEXIBILITY FOCUS** | | | |
| Standing chest expansion with forward fold | | • Hold for 3-5 breaths. | Page 130 |
| Kneeling shoulder stretch | | • Hold for 5-10 breaths. | Page 192 |
| Camel | | • Hold for 5-10 breaths. | Page 148 |

Additional practice
• Perform standing balance poses, such as tree, eagle, and balancing half moon (see chapter 6).

# Five-Minute Poststretch for Any Sport

Any athlete or gym-goer can use this well-rounded stretch following any physical activity. Hold each pose for 5 to 10 breaths (or 5 to 10 breaths on each side, when applicable). See chapter 9 for information on stretching regularly for strength, balance, and flexibility. This workout relieves stress and tension in the lower back, hips, hamstrings, and hip flexors.

YogaFit may improve your performance in your sport, reduce your risk of injury, and will add to your overall enjoyment.

| Child's pose | | • Hold for 5-10 breaths, focusing on deep breaths. | Page 184 |
|---|---|---|---|
| Rabbit | | • Breathe deeply into the back.<br>• Keep weight off the head.<br>• Hold for 5-10 breaths. | Page 222 |
| Seated spinal twist or half lord of the fishes | *or* | • Inhale and lengthen; exhale and rotate.<br>• Use your core versus your arm to deepen rotation.<br>• For half lord of the fishes fold legs so thighs relax down toward floor.<br>• Maintain lengthened spine into the twist.<br>• Switch sides.<br>• Hold for 5-10 breaths. | Pages 172 and 174 |
| Butterfly | | • Hold butterfly for 5-10 breaths.<br>• Lie on your back with the soles of your feet together, knees open wide for 5-10 breaths.<br>• Relax completely. | Page 200 |
| Knees to chest | | • Place hands on your hamstrings versus your shins.<br>• Focus on releasing your lower back.<br>• Hold for 5-10 breaths. | Page 208 |
| Supine half lotus | | • Relax completely.<br>• Avoid any position that causes discomfort in the knee.<br>• Switch sides.<br>• Hold for 5-10 breaths. | Page 206 |

| | | | |
|---|---|---|---|
| **Big toe hold** | | • Keep both hips on the mat, bending knees as necessary.<br>• Switch sides.<br>• Hold each phase for 5 breaths. | Page 212 |
| **Upside-down pigeon** | | • Flex your feet.<br>• Switch sides.<br>• Hold for 5-10 breaths. | Page 204 |
| **Bridge or wheel** | *or* | • Practice expanding breath.<br>• Slide your shoulders away from your ears.<br>• Follow with knees to chest (page 208).<br>• Hold for 5-10 breaths. | Pages 154 and 156 |
| **Dead bug** | | • Keep your tailbone on the floor.<br>• Stack your ankles over your knees.<br>• Hold for 5-10 breaths. | Page 210 |
| **Fish** | | • Follows inversions as a counterpose to open throat and chest.<br>• Hold for 5-10 breaths. | Page 220 |
| **Knees to chest** | | • Place hands on your hamstrings, not your shins.<br>• Focus on releasing your lower back.<br>• Hold for 5-10 breaths. | Page 208 |
| **Supine spinal twist** | | • Keeping shoulders relaxed to floor, supporting leg as needed. Push through the heel of the straight leg.<br>• Hold for 5-10 breaths each side. | Page 178 |
| **Final relaxation** | | • Find a comfortable position that allows you to relax. (Option: place feet on floor with knees bent.)<br>• Let go of distractions.<br>• Let go of controlling your breath.<br>• Hold for as long as time allows. | Page 228 |

CHAPTER

# Yoga as Therapy

Yoga therapy is about using yogic tools to increase wellness, result-ing in optimal health and balance, or to help heal from an injury or an illness. Unlike the Western medical system, yoga therapy takes an integrative approach, seeing the whole person and not just the affected part. Yoga differs from traditional exercise because of the mindful aspect of the practice. Mindfulness helps you derive some of the benefits of practicing yoga. The attention to breath is also a key factor, and so are the multiplanar movements of a single practice. This chapter explores how yoga can help heal both the body and the mind.

All yoga is therapy at some level. Yoga helps you decrease stress and the associated secretion of stress hormones, including cortisol. Stress is a factor in almost every disease-plaguing society today. Stress lowers the immune system, affecting physical health as well as emotional and mental well-being. Chronic stress is linked to high blood pressure, sleep disturbances, obesity, gastrointestinal problems such as irritable bowel syndrome, depression, skin disorders, decreased memory, headaches, and more.

Stress comes in two forms, eustress and distress. The Greek prefix *eu-* means "well" or "good." The term describes the kind of stress that motivates you to accomplish things. How you perceive challenges will determine the physiological response of the body. Each person perceives and handles life's challenges differently, and one person's *eu*stress can be another person's *dis*tress. The body responds to a threat (distress) by activating the autonomic nervous system, more specifically the sympathetic nervous system known as the fight-or-flight response to secrete hormones that prepare the body to deal with the threat. The sympathetic nervous system is important for survival in the presence of a threat. The problem comes when the stress becomes chronic, either through actual physical circumstances or perception, and the brain and body are continuously in a state of arousal. The body has to work harder to maintain homeostasis (balance in the body systems). Continued exposure to cortisol and other stress hormones damages the brain and nervous system, and the result over time can be stress-related disease. Yoga provides you with the tools to elicit the relaxation response (activating the parasympathetic nervous system), thus turning off the stress response. It can also help you shift your perception of events.

Yoga affects all layers of your being (koshas), giving you several ways to practice both on and off the mat. Practicing even one of the eight limbs (yamas, niyamas, asana, pranayama, pratyahara, dharana, dhyana, samadhi; see chapter 1) has the potential to have a profound positive impact on your health. You can think of the yamas and niyamas as guideposts for navigating perception of life circumstances with increased mindfulness. Asana (the physical practice of yoga poses) keeps the body healthy, strong, and flexible. Pranayama (breath practices) helps increase vitality and mindfulness of the breath. Simply taking a deeper breath helps bring more balance to your autonomic nervous system by activating the vagal system (part of the nervous system that links body and brain). Practicing the limbs of pratyahara, dharana, and dhyana helps you stay focused even when distractions are present. Increasing mindfulness enhances the health and function of the body and the brain. Depending on the type of meditation practiced, changes happen in various areas of the brain including an increase in volume of brain tissue and rewiring and activation in areas of the brain that helps us become less reactive to distractions and stressors and increase feelings of well-being and happiness. Chapter 12 discusses meditation in more detail.

Healing results from the process of *going in* rather than the practice of doing poses. In terms of healing, *how* you practice yoga has much more to do with the outcome than *what* you practice. Your practice on the mat is just one of the ways to a more balanced system. Yoga has many paths that can lead toward healing. Among these paths of yoga are hatha (physical), bhakti (devotion), raja (meditation), and karma (selfless service). The yoga practice described in this book is a vinyasa (flowing) style of hatha yoga. This style can certainly be included in a healing practice, but in times of injury or illness YogaFit suggests shifting to a more restorative practice. Restorative yoga is more restful yet can still be an active practice. Commonly, restorative yoga is practiced with several props with the intention of supporting the pose so that all tension is dissolved and the practitioner can fully relax the body and the mind. However, if you don't have the props available, consider other ways to make a pose more restorative.

## Purpose of Restorative Yoga

Restorative yoga is designed to heal and restore the health and vitality of the mind and body. Throughout the years, practitioners have been using restorative yoga and its many healing poses for a variety of conditions, including back pain, neck pain, high or low blood pressure, infertility, migraines, asthma, autoimmune disorders, and chronic fatigue.

The intention of restorative yoga is to trigger exactly the things that are ailing you while also alleviating any stress that you face in your practice. For instance, if you are straining to keep the body in a pose, then the practice becomes counterproductive to the healing process because it elicits a stress response.

This is where the use of props can be helpful to support a pose. Props such as YogaFit egg blocks, rectangular blocks, straps, chairs, bolsters, foam wedges, sandbags, and core balls can completely support the body as it rests for a period of time in a healing position, so you can simply focus on breathing as you restore vitality to the body and the mind.

# Purpose of Using Props

Using props to explore your yoga practice enables you to modify poses physically while maintaining the maximum health benefits in a posture. Review the various props available in chapter 2.

Although many studios use props today, they are a fairly new enhancement to the hatha practice and its traditional asanas. The Iyengar style of hatha yoga uses props in order to help you experience poses in appropriate alignment and without stress, so that you can be free of distractions and achieve unity in the body and mind.

In its purest form, the Iyengar style of yoga involves very little vinyasa; it does not focus on linking poses together in unity with specific breathing patterns. In Iyengar yoga, once poses are in perfect alignment, they are held for a prolonged time in an effort to build muscle memory while reaping the physical and mental benefits from the posture.

Although it is possible to do yoga without props, they help to create an ideal alignment specific to each person's body type, physical history, and psychological response. In the Iyengar tradition, props enable you to create more physical balance in the body so that you may experience a reflection of that balance in your mind.

The use of props allows people with hesitancy, tightness, balance problems, stiffness, or other special needs to practice with security, confidence, and safety. Often people are unable to take advantage of the benefits of yoga because of these factors; working with props will generally serve this type of person.

In some poses, props help you to completely release and relax; in others, they help you build strength and balance in the body. Practicing yoga with challenges and imbalances can sometimes be unsafe. However, with the aid of props, you begin to experience the benefits of a pose as well as understand how the pose is supposed to feel, imprinting that feeling in your muscle memory.

Yoga allows natural freedom of movement to be restored, and strength to be regenerated. Yoga exercise must work *with* the body, not against it. Each pose offers a way of releasing stress and tension, and restorative yoga helps guide you through your practice in a stress-free way.

YogaFit teachers work both with props and without props. In the case where no props are available, they instead change the pose to fit the body. Teachers practice with the YogaFit essence in mind, remembering that no perfect expression of a pose exists and that the journey into and out of the pose is what matters. For example, in forward fold, you are encouraged to bend the knees in order to take pressure off the back. Just this simple change enables someone with tighter hamstrings to breathe more deeply and protect the low back while stretching the hamstrings. If you are straining to get into a particular version of a pose, then you are creating muscle tension and stimulating the sympathetic nervous system. Instead, create a practice that helps you elicit the relaxation response (parasympathetic nervous system) so that more healing can take place.

## Creating a Restorative Therapeutic Practice

The YogaFit essence is *breathing, feeling, and listening to your body; letting go of expectations, judgments, and competition; and staying in the present moment.*

When you are working to heal injury or illness or even just to correct posture, no one set routine will work for everyone. Choose poses that feel good for the body. If you find a position that is painful, come out of it immediately. Using the YogaFit essence as your guide, modify your positions as needed. If you slow down and listen to your body, feeling your way into a pose, then you have less chance of getting injured. Releasing any expectations about the way a particular pose is supposed to look can also help you create more movement at each joint. When using yoga as therapy, be less concerned about creating poses and more concerned about creating pain-free movement while paying attention to and studying your default habits. Slowing down your practice and movements can help to increase your awareness. Sometimes people move in exercise or in daily life in unconscious patterns that may be doing more harm than good. An example would be trying to move into triangle pose using someone else or a picture as a guide. If you place the hand too close to the floor, you may move beyond a safe range of motion for your body or compensate in other areas of the body.

A restorative therapeutic practice can be either active or passive. The key is to pay attention to each moment and notice how your body is responding. As you move into a pose, do you move easily and keep a deep, slow, smooth breath, or do you notice a catch or a rough spot in the transition? Do you notice tension anywhere in the body as you move into and out of or hold a pose? Answers to these questions are clues to how our nervous system is reacting to your practice. The goal is to maintain a relaxed state in both the body and the mind throughout the practice.

# Restorative Therapeutics: Active and Passive Poses

The following poses are some examples of how to create a more therapeutic expression of certain poses, even standing poses. In the active poses the theme is *less is more*. You can apply this principle to any pose you choose. Pay attention to the breath and the movement of the joints. In any of the propped poses, you can use rectangular blocks or blankets if egg blocks are not available. Keep in mind that the following are just suggestions, so play around with your poses and see what feels good for your body. If any pose creates pain or discomfort, adjust your position so that you can be in it safely and without tension.

## Triangle With Hand on Thigh or Shin

Move into triangle pose, and pay special attention to keeping the spine in neutral and the bandhas active as you move at the hip joint only. Keep the breath full and deep, and notice if you are tempted to move the torso to reach the hand further down the leg. Alternatively, you could use a block or a chair for the lower hand to rest on, but the idea here is to notice how much hip movement we have while keeping the spine in neutral and the chest open. See chapter 6 for the triangle pose.

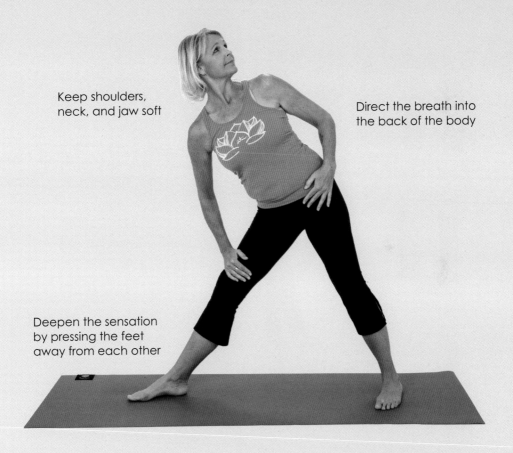

Keep shoulders, neck, and jaw soft

Direct the breath into the back of the body

Deepen the sensation by pressing the feet away from each other

# Downward-Facing Dog on the Wall

Facing a wall, hinge at the hips while walking your hands down the wall until the hips are at 90 degrees with the feet stacked under the hips. Bend the knees as needed in order to keep the spine in neutral alignment (the back will be flat). Energize the pose by pushing into the feet (pada bandha) and the hands (hasta bandha) and activating the core. Reach the heart center toward the wall, and breathe deeply and easily. See chapter 7 for the downward-facing dog pose.

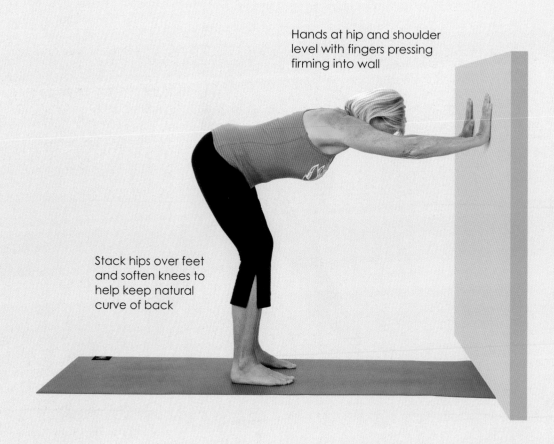

Hands at hip and shoulder level with fingers pressing firming into wall

Stack hips over feet and soften knees to help keep natural curve of back

# Downward-Facing Dog With Egg Blocks

Using the egg blocks helps create a grounding sensation in the pose. The eggs work well to fill in the space because they contour to the arches. The eggs can be placed against the wall if preferred for additional support. Bend the knees as needed to keep the spine long and to take stress out of the shoulders. See chapter 7 for the downward-facing dog pose.

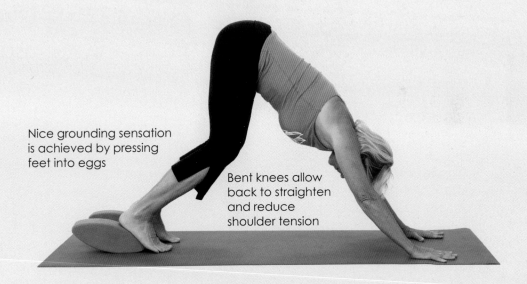

Nice grounding sensation is achieved by pressing feet into eggs

Bent knees allow back to straighten and reduce shoulder tension

# Twisting Chair—Gentle

This is a gentle version of twisting chair, focusing on the movement of the spine and the shoulder girdle. Keep the knees in line with each other as you twist to one side on the exhalation. Hold for 3 to 5 breaths, and repeat to the other side. The idea is to create rotational mobility in the spine in this pose, letting go of the need to twist too far. Check in with the breath and make sure it's full and easy. See chapter 8 for the twisting chair pose.

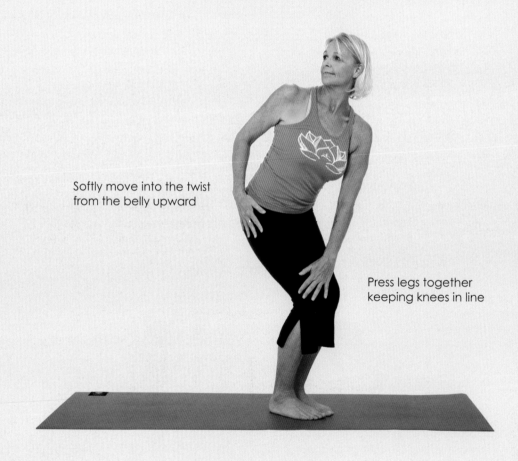

Softly move into the twist from the belly upward

Press legs together keeping knees in line

# Supported Cobra, Sphinx, and Locust

These energizing poses use the egg blocks to reinforce the idea of lengthening the spine forward in either pose. Place the egg blocks under the chest, and reach the heart center forward. For cobra pose, keep the lower body on the floor while lifting the upper body as high as comfortable. For sphinx pose, place the forearms on the mat and press into the mat while reaching the chest center forward. For locust pose, lift the upper body and the lower body. See chapter 5 for the cobra pose and chapter 7 for the locust pose.

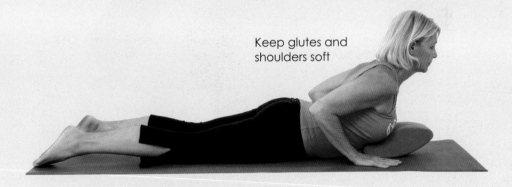

Reaching forward with your head over the eggs encourages a gentle lengthening of the spine

Keep glutes and shoulders soft

From legs up the wall pose, place the feet hip-width apart on the wall and lift the hips, placing the hands on the back or placing a bolster, blanket, or egg blocks to support the hip and lower back. Walk the shoulder blades together, breathing expansively into the lungs. Press your feet firmly into the wall. Stay here for 3 to 5 minutes, and lower back down into legs up the wall pose. Avoid this pose if you have upper-back or neck injury or pain. See chapter 9 for the shoulderstand pose.

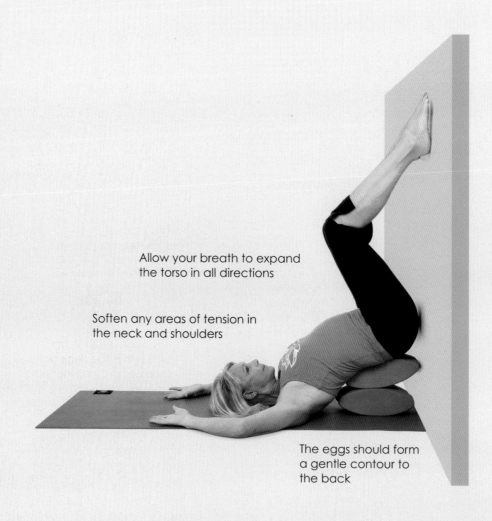

Allow your breath to expand the torso in all directions

Soften any areas of tension in the neck and shoulders

The eggs should form a gentle contour to the back

# Heart Opener on Egg Blocks (Supported Fish)

Lie back on two egg blocks so that they support the lower back. Place a third egg under the head to level the chin. The arms can rest out to the sides or on the belly, whichever is more comfortable. Stay here for 5 to 10 minutes while using an easy, comfortable breath. See chapter 9 for the fish pose.

For more relaxation, place the feet further apart and let the feet and legs roll out

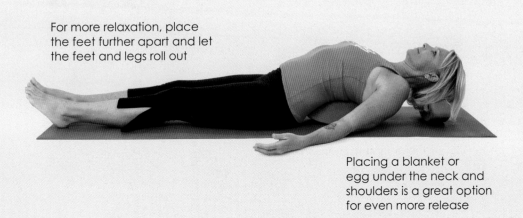

Placing a blanket or egg under the neck and shoulders is a great option for even more release

# Reclining Butterfly

Lie on your back with the feet together and a comfortable distance from the hips. Relax the legs open, and place the egg blocks under the thighs as pictured for support. You can also use a blanket or rectangular blocks. Stay here for 5 to 10 minutes while breathing into the belly and extending the exhalations if comfortable. See chapter 9 for the butterfly pose.

Breathe into the expanse of the torso and exhale slowly melting through the hips

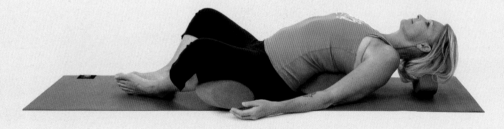

# Bridge on a Block

From bridge pose, lower your hips down onto an egg. Gently rock if your egg is placed on the rounded side. See chapter 7 for the bridge pose.

Consciously soften the pelvis

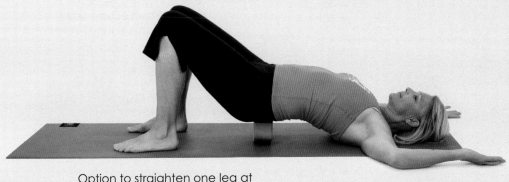

Option to straighten one leg at a time to bring more sensation into the front of the hip

# Prone Twist on Bolster

Place egg blocks end to end in the center of the mat. For added comfort, place a folded blanket over the blocks. With your thighs perpendicular across the mat, place your hands on either side of the blocks and elongate the spine. Slowly lower down over the blocks. The head can either be facing the direction of the knees or the opposite direction for more sensation. Stay here for 5 to 10 minutes, and repeat to the other side. See chapter 8 for the supine spinal twist pose.

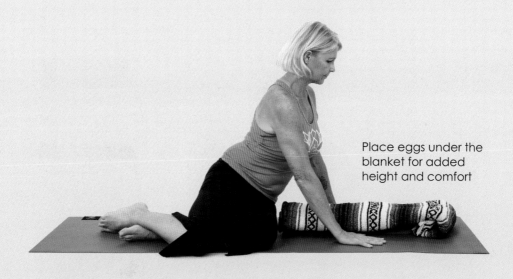

Place eggs under the blanket for added height and comfort

Relax and let go

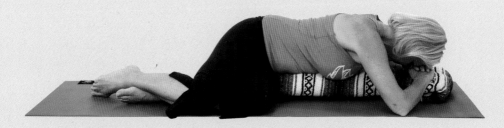

# Legs Up the Wall Supported With Eggs

Place egg blocks under the low back to provide a nice support for the spine. See chapter 9 for the legs up the wall pose.

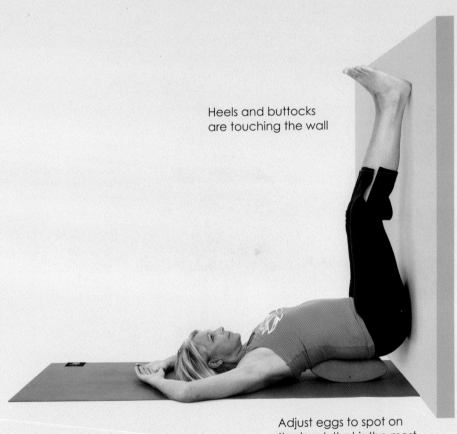

Heels and buttocks are touching the wall

Adjust eggs to spot on the back that is the most comfortable for you

**YogaFit for Warriors**

YogaFit for Warriors is a special trauma-sensitive YogaFit format that addresses the growing needs of the U.S. military. Both veterans and active duty suicide rates have been alarmingly high over the last few years. The United States has been in a state of ongoing wars for over 15 years, and people in the military community (active duty, spouses, children, extended family, and support staff) are all impacted as is the entire nation. YogaFit for Warriors was originally conceived out of a desire to bring the healing practice of yoga and meditation to America's military community as well as to increase awareness of the plight of the U.S. military and their families. However, stress is not unique to the military, and the program has grown to encompass people from all walks of life who are feeling the effects of chronic stress. As a somatic treatment, yoga works to heal the body from stored trauma and the damage it creates. To find trainings in your area, please go to www.yogafit.com/trainings/100-hour-warriors-program. These trainings are open to anyone.

Posttraumatic stress disorder (PTSD) can result from being involved in or exposed to a traumatic event or a series of events. It is characterized by flashbacks, nightmares, feeling isolated and numb, being easily triggered and explosive, difficulty sleeping, among other symptoms. When a person has PTSD, the mind and body become "stuck" at the time that the lower-level brain kicked in to fight, flee, or freeze. When attempting to heal from a traumatic experience, traditional therapies focus mainly on top–down (called cognitive) approaches to healing trauma by examining behaviors from a standpoint of logic and understanding. However, experts are recognizing that trauma does indeed get stuck in the neural pathways activated by the primitive brain, and no amount of mental health therapy will help the person get fully "unstuck."

YogaFit is committed to raising awareness of the symptoms of PTSD and helping as many people toward the healing path of a simple mindful YogaFit practice. These are the six YogaFit Warrior trainings:

- YogaFit for Warriors
- Healing Emotional and Physical Trauma
- Restorative Therapeutics: The Art and Science of Healing
- Mood Balancing
- YogaFit for Addictions and Recovery
- YogaFit Warriors for Kids

The YogaFit for Warriors trainings are open to anyone who wants to find out more about how to create a healing practice. After taking the trainings, instructors understand how to create a healing and transformational environment for anyone dealing with chronic stress or PTSD. For those who are taking it for personal reasons, they will have a practice firmly in place for their own use.

Yoga sets up a safe environment that enables a person suffering from PTSD to become reacquainted with his or her body and emotions and begin the healing process. The process of healing involves regaining trust in a body that has become an enemy of sorts, because it is filled with pain. In a carefully crafted yoga practice, a person can practice letting down his or her guard and begin to heal the nervous system's communication by developing the ability stay in that relaxed state of healing for increasingly longer periods of time.

Find out more about YogaFit for Warriors at yogafit.com/trainings/100-hour-warriors-program.

CHAPTER  12

# Benefits of Meditation

The ancient yogic texts describe the goal of yoga as unification of the body and the mind and spirit and also realization of the connection between all life. The Satchidananda quote on this page is the second sutra (sutra means thread) in the ancient text of raja yoga. Raja yoga is known as the path of meditation. The sutra is explaining that if we can quiet the chatter in our mind or be nonreactive to it and stay focused, we have reached our goal in yoga. Meditation can simply be thought of focusing on one thing, such as the breath, for a period of time. When practiced regularly, meditation can bring wonderful health benefits and help you manage your stress levels. Meditation is about turning inward, observing your habits, and increasing your awareness, leading you away from reactivity and toward more mindfulness.

> Sutra 1.2: "Yogas chitta vrtti nirodha" (The restraint of the modifications of the mind-stuff is yoga; Satchidananda, 1990, p. 3)

Much of people's daily life is spent in their heads, focused on what they're thinking rather than on what they're sensing or feeling. People are bombarded daily with information and stimuli that they must sort through and process. With all the demands of work and home, people are often required to stay one mental step ahead just to get through the day. The problem is that when you navigate through life led by your thoughts alone, you miss out on a world of information available to you through your body and spirit. Yogic philosophy states that suffering comes from your thoughts and from a disconnection from the greater universe. Think about how many times you created a story in your head, which then created anxiety or negative shift in mood. It happens on a daily basis unless you are mindful about your daily thoughts and habits. Daily habits of thought, word, and actions shape you. You create your universe. If you are constantly thinking negative thoughts, your nervous system responds by activating the stress response. When you are subjected to chronic stress, a shift occurs in the balance of the autonomic nervous system and in how the brain processes information. If your fight-or-flight nervous system is chronically on, the resulting flood of stress hormones damages the brain structures and shuts off the pathway that sends body sense information to the brain. Yoga and meditation tune up your nervous system, and they balance and strengthen the connections between the body and the mind.

The ancient practice of meditation is as integral to yoga as the poses are, and they have the same intention: not to tune out, but to tune *in* to a frequency that is long forgotten or perhaps undiscovered. To meditate is to become acutely aware of what is going on within you. It's about learning to tame your mind so that you can focus all your energy and awareness on the task at hand. The practice of meditation helps you stay centered regardless of your circumstances. It doesn't teach you to avoid pain or discomfort but to experience and accept it so that you can move through any situation with profound clarity and a sense of inner peace and calm. Meditation is a wonderful way to tap into your internal sense of knowing and stay in touch with your eternal essence.

At first, meditation can be awkward and unfamiliar. These feelings are common, and they are natural. It might be eye-opening to discover that you are controlled by incessant thoughts, and it might be frustrating to realize that many of them are unnecessary and perhaps even based in misperception or falsehood. Sitting in silence, you might realize how many common distractions compete for your attention, including doubt, sleepiness, and restlessness. Rather than using up even more energy in fighting these hindrances, you eventually realize it's far easier to acknowledge them and release them. Distractions will never let up, but you can teach yourself to let them go. In fact, an awareness of your thoughts and distractions is the first step toward developing a successful meditation practice that will improve your physical and mental well-being.

When you refine your ability to slip into a state of awareness and being, you can bring this focus into other areas of your life. No matter what's happening in your immediate environment, you can step back and respond rather than react. Whether it's an athletic competition, work, a difficult conversation, or a game you're playing, you will enjoy what you're doing much more, and perhaps you'll even do it much better.

Give yourself permission to be a beginner, and know that with practice your ability to concentrate will improve. Eventually, you'll find that during meditation you might slip between thoughts, or you might discover yourself

**You are not seeking to find anything through the practice of meditation. Rather, it is through meditation that you are found. It's a mistake to think that through meditation you are trying to become somebody else. The true intent of yoga and meditation is to become the best possible version of yourself.**

unaware of any thoughts at all. In this place, you might not only lose track of what you hear around you but discover you've lost all sense of time. With practice, you'll find that you can meditate in a noisy airport or on a busy street corner without becoming distracted.

# Benefits of Meditation

Because practicing meditation helps you to slow your breath, quiet your mind, and find peace, it can be beneficial physically, mentally, and emotionally. Meditation is now commonly used to treat mental health disorders, addiction, and everyday stress, as well as to heal physical ailments and promote better sleep.

**Physical Benefits**

- It stimulates your parasympathetic nervous system, the branch of your peripheral nervous system that helps your body return to a calm, relaxed state after the threat of danger, or even daily stress, has passed. When this branch is activated, your body can naturally rejuvenate, repair, and rebuild itself.
- It reduces blood pressure, blood glucose levels, and cholesterol levels—all factors in cardiovascular disease.
- It clears your mind for better quality sleep.
- It improves athletic performance by refining your ability to focus on a goal or situation (another term for meditation used in this way is visualization).
- It slows your respiration for longer, deeper breaths.
- It boosts your immune system by slowing the production of the stress hormone cortisol.
- It increases cortical thickness in the brain, resulting in increased cognitive function and memory.
- It increases the enzyme telomerase, which protects the ends of the DNA called telomeres resulting in an increase in cellular longevity.

**Mental and Emotional Benefits**

- It reduces anxiety and depression by enabling your body to balance its own neurochemical system.
- It allows you to make better decisions and improve critical thinking.
- It breaks unhealthy habits by helping you detach emotions associated with an action from the action itself.
- It improves communication with yourself. When you better understand your thought processes, you have more control over what you think.
- It helps you shift to a more positive outlook on life by activating the left prefrontal cortex in the brain, the area responsible for feelings of contentment and self-worth.

- It helps you stay in the present moment. When you let go of the past and the future, you live 100 percent in the now, which affects all aspects of your life and relationships.

# Active Meditation Techniques

Earlier in the chapter, meditation was described as simply focusing on a single thing, such as the breath, for a period of time. Traditionally, the physical postures were introduced to prepare the body for sitting in meditation for extended periods of time. Although over time, the physical practice makes it easier to sit for longer periods of time, you don't have to be sitting down or be still to be successfully meditating. Many meditation traditions and techniques exist. Westerners, accustomed to fast-paced living and constant information exchange, often benefit more from active meditation techniques. Active meditation involves focusing your thoughts and awareness on a particular thought, idea, visualization, or concept. Choosing to focus on something positive can help you rid your mind of negative thoughts and emotions and other clutter. If you aren't comfortable sitting on the floor, choose a chair. Or, choose a walking or standing meditation. You can even meditate during your physical yoga practice or any other exercise or activity. Whatever your meditation practice looks like, be sure to embrace this YogaFit essence: *Let go of all judgment of your experience.*

Here are some steps to help you establish a personal active meditation practice:

1. When you begin, commit to meditating at least 5 minutes every day (more, if possible; later, you can add minutes). Set an alarm or timer so that you don't have to keep an eye on the clock. To help make your meditation practice a habit, practice at the same time each day, or establish a routine, such as meditating immediately after your YogaFit session. Finally, if you have room, establish a special place to sit and meditate at home. Place a chair in a corner near a favorite window, or surround a cushion with your favorite candles. Create your own sacred space. Knowing you have somewhere you love to go will help you get there.

2. Whether you're in a chair, on a cushion, or on the floor, sit comfortably with your spine straight. A straight (neutral) spine is important for breathing with ease, facilitating energy flow and circulation throughout the body as well as keeping muscle tension at bay. If you're not comfortable, you'll be distracted. If you're practicing before or after your YogaFit workout, roll up your mat and sit on it; elevating your hips eases tension in your hips and hamstrings and improves circulation to your legs.

3. Use the relaxation breath technique (see chapter 3). Sit upright with a neutral spine, relax your abdomen, and breathe quietly without forcing your exhalations. Take the same amount of time for your inhalation and your exhalation, consciously beginning your inhalation just as your exhalation ends.

Your abdominal muscles must not be constrained by tension or clothing; you must be completely free to move.

4. Select one of the following techniques. If the technique you choose doesn't work, let it go and try another. In any of these techniques, choosing an intention of gratitude can enhance your practice and help you feel the positive effects faster. Many studies support the expression of gratitude and appreciation with positive physical and mental health outcomes, including a greater feeling of connection to the world around you.

- Choose a mantra (word or phrase), thought, or feeling on which to meditate. Repeat your mantra over and over in rhythm with your breath. You can repeat the mantra out loud or silently if you prefer. If your first choice leads to negative thoughts or feelings, let it go and choose something else. For example, a common mantra is "om" (pronounced *aaaaaooooommmmm*), which represents the root of all sounds that are ever-present as vibrations in your body.

- Visualize a person, object, or place in which you find peace, love, or gratitude, such as a lotus blossom, pet, loved one, or a quiet beach.

- If preparing for a performance or competition, visualize yourself succeeding; use all your senses as you mentally act out the scenario. Appreciate your talents such as strength, speed, and agility.

- Use a guided meditation. Many such meditations are available on CD or as part of meditation apps. Relax, and fully listen to each word.

- Use an affirmation card with a phrase that inspires or strengthens you. Many books and box sets with positive affirmations are available. Or you can make your own. Examples include *I am at peace* and *I am love.*

- Focus on a small, meaningful object held in your hand or placed in front you. Use a mala, rosary, or worry beads as a counting tool to help give a focal point for attention in both the body and the mind. A set of beads can help keep the count of a mantra during meditation if your desire is to engage in a set number of repetitions.

- Make your food a meditation practice. Eat slowly and with full appreciation for the food. Focus on the texture, taste, smell, and appearance of the food. (This practice is especially fun with chocolate!)

- If sitting still is too challenging, try a walking meditation. Walk slowly with intention to notice every step. Focus on the movement of each body part and the feel of the feet as they touch the ground. Be very aware of the sights and sounds surrounding you. You can count your steps as a way to stay focused.

5. Keep a gratitude journal. Writing is a wonderful form of meditation. Each day, write five or six things that you are grateful for. After meditating, reflect on the experience in a journal. For example, write down any techniques you tried and what you experienced practicing them. What were your thoughts and feelings before, during, and after meditating? Also note whether you made

any headway toward working out questions or situations you've struggled to resolve. Finally, keep track of the benefits you notice from incorporating meditation into your yoga practice. These notes will become incentives to continue.

# Recognizing Your Success

How do you know if you're meditating successfully? People describe their meditative states in a wide variety of ways. Some see a single source of light, some see themselves from a distance, and others see images or even sense colors. Some people see or feel nothing they can express in words. Some experience a wonderful state of *being-ness,* an inner glow of warmth and peace. All these experiences indicate a successful meditation session. Just as there's no best version of a yoga pose, there's no one best way to meditate.

As you explore the meditation techniques described in this chapter, remember that every day is different and every session is different; you're constantly faced with new struggles and challenges. Yet your inner truths remain the same; you need only to look within. Whatever your meditation looks or feels like, remember to embrace the essence of YogaFit and let go of all expectations. Take a moment now to commit to a daily meditation practice for the next 30 days following these simple guidelines:

- Choose a time of day (whatever works best for you, but it is recommended you choose the same time each day for consistency).
- Choose how many minutes each day (start with 5 minutes and then add time as you feel comfortable). One suggestion is to add 5 minutes each week so that by the fourth week you will be meditating 20 minutes each day.
- Choose a technique that appeals to you (remember you can meditate sitting down or during movement). If you will be sitting down to meditate, create a special meditation space with pillows and perhaps flowers, a special trinket or photo, and other items that make it inviting.
- Journal for a few minutes after each session. At the end of 30 days recommit to another 30 days and perhaps try a different form or use with the same technique if it worked well.

# Chakras

The word *chakra* is Sanskrit for "wheel" or "disk." Seven chakra energy centers (nerve bundles) exist along the spinal column, as shown in the figure on this page. Each of these centers correlates to major nerve ganglia branching forth from the spinal column and has a corresponding relationship to one of the glands of the body's endocrine system. Each chakra stimulates different organs and systems in the body. The first six chakras begin at the coccyx and continue up to the cervical vertebrae, while the seventh chakra is associated with the cerebral cortex of the brain. The chakras are part of your pranamaya kosha (energy layer), and they interact with all the other layers of your being (see discussion of koshas in chapter 1).

| Spinal Column/Nerves | Seven Chakras/Nerve Bundles | YogaFit Energy Centers |
|---|---|---|
| | Chakra Seven – Cerebral Cortex | Crown Center |
| | Chakra Six – Carotid Plexus | Brow Center |
| | Chakra Five – Pharyngeal Plexus | Throat Center |
| | Chakra Four – Pulmonary and Cardiac Plexus | Heart Center |
| | Chakra Three – Solar Plexus | Solar Plexus Center |
| | Chakra Two – Sacral Plexus | Navel Center |
| | Chakra One – Coccygeal Plexus | Root Center |

Hatha yoga exercises, such as the ones used in YogaFit, activate these energy centers by their very nature to enhance overall balance and performance. Moving the spine keeps the nerve impulses flowing. The following warm-up and workout formats are designed to target the seven chakras in your body to help them function correctly and prevent nerve bundles from getting blocked. Traditionally, the chakras are also associated with various issues and concepts associated with mental, emotional, and spiritual life. The following chart serves as a brief and general introduction to these associations. It also indicates each chakra's corresponding color. To learn more about the chakras and how they relate to you, order YogaFit's *Chakra Balancing* listed in the Recommended Reading and Shopping section of appendix B.

## YogaFit Chakra Energy Warm-Up

| | |
|---|---|
| **First chakra** | Moonflowers |
| **Second chakra** | Sunflowers |
| **Third chakra** | Chair flow (described in standard standing warm-up and standard lying-down warm-up in chapter 10) |
| **Fourth chakra** | Cat and cow (described in standard standing warm-up and standard lying-down warm-up in chapter 10) |
| **Fifth chakra** | Plank push-up series (described in the flex and flow workout in chapter 10) |
| **Sixth chakra** | Modified flow series |
| **Seventh chakra** | Spinal balance (described in standard standing warm-up and standard lying-down warm-up in chapter 10) |

## YogaFit Chakra Energy Workout

| Chakra name | Physical focus | Mental, emotional, and spiritual focus | Color visualization |
|---|---|---|---|
| 1. Root | Mountain pose and breathing (see chapter 3) | Grounding | Red |
| 2. Navel | Flow sequences | Creativity, flow, and sensuality | Orange |
| 3. Solar plexus | Mountain II poses, such as warrior I, warrior II, warrior III, and reverse warrior | Discipline, willpower, personal power | Yellow |
| 4. Heart | Expansion poses, such as camel, standing backbend, and chest expansion with forward fold | Love, self-acceptance, agape, openness | Green |
| 5. Throat | Poses such as incline plank and shoulderstand; chanting or mantras (see chapter 12) | Communication | Blue |
| 6. Third eye | Balancing poses; creative visualization (see chapter 12) | Insight or vision | Purple |
| 7. Crown | Final relaxation; meditation (see chapter 12) | Unification with higher self and universe | White |

# Recommended Reading and Shopping

I have selected a variety of books and other tools to broaden your understanding of yoga and other related mind–body topics. To order the books listed here or for more titles, visit our website at www.yogafit.com or visit www.amazon.com.

- *Yoga as Medicine: The Yogic Prescription for Health and Healing*, Timothy McCall
- *Anatomy and Asana: Preventing Yoga Injuries*, Susi Hately Aldous
- *Chakra Meditation: Discover Energy, Creativity Focus, Love Communication, Wisdom, and Spirit*, Swami Saradananda
- *Chakra Balancing*, Judith Anodea
- *Creative Visualization: Use the Power of Your Imagination to Create What You Want in Your Life* (book and workbook), Shakti Gawain
- *Eating Mindfully: How to End Mindless Eating and Enjoy a Balanced Relationship with Food*, Susan Albers
- *Natural Prozac*, Joel C. Robertson
- *Pathways to Joy: The Master Vivekananda on the Four Yoga Paths to God*, Swami Vivekananda and Dave Deluca
- *Practicing the Power of Now*, Eckhart Tolle
- *The Key Muscles of Yoga*, Ray Long
- *The Language of Yoga: Complete A to Y Guide to Asana Names, Sanskrit Terms, and Chants*, Nicolai Bachman
- *The Living Gita*, Sri Swami Satchidananda
- *The Mandala of Being: Discovering the Power of Awareness*, Richard Moss, MD
- *The Yoga Sutras of Patanjali*, Sri Swami Satchidananda
- *Your Body Speaks Your Mind*, Deb Shapiro
- *Growing the Positive Mind*, William K. Larkin

- *YogaLean*, Beth Shaw
- *Overcoming Trauma Through Yoga: Reclaiming Your Body*, David Emerson and Elizabeth Hopper, PhD
- *In an Unspoken Voice: How The Body Releases Trauma and Restores Goodness*, Peter Levine
- *The Subtle Body: An Encyclopedia of your Energetic Anatomy*, Cyndi Dale
- *Clutter Busting Your Life: Clearing Physical and Emotional Clutter to Reconnect with Yourself and Others*, Brooks Palmer
- *Emotional Healing with Essential Oils*, Daniel Macdonald
- *Yoga of Heart: The Healing Power of Intimate Connection*, Mark Whitwell
- *Yoga for Depression: A Compassionate Guide to Relieve Suffering Through Yoga*, Amy Weintraub
- *The Woman's Book of Yoga and Health: A Lifelong Guide to Wellness*, Linda Sparrowe and Patricia Walden
- *Relax and Renew: Restful Yoga for Stressful Times*, Judith Hanson Lasater, PhD

YogaFit continues to produce DVDs for every level, from *YogaFit Beginners* to *Active Advanced*, as well as DVDs for specialty populations, including *YogaFit Plus* for larger bodies, *YogaFit Seniors*, *YogaFit Kids*, and *YogaFit Prenatal*. To order or to get more information on which formats are most appropriate for you, visit our website at www.yogafit.com.

YogaFit also provides CDs to enhance your YogaFit experience. Our *Active, SlowFlow,* and *Zen Series* CDs are compiled to correspond with the three mountains of warm-up, work, and cool-down. The collection includes a variety of artists and styles, that you can find the perfect music for your practice or class. To order, listen to CDs, or find out more about which formats are most appropriate for you, visit our website at www.yogafit.com.

Since its inception, YogaFit has offered high-quality, high-performance clothing and accessories at competitive prices. Bulk pricing is available on all YogaFit products. Just order a minimum of 12 pieces (per style) or items to receive incredible savings. To order or view photographs of our clothing line, as well as our mats, blocks, straps, and more, visit www.yogafit.com.

# YogaFit Teacher Training and Partner Programs

YogaFit is committed to providing you with the best educational and business opportunities to further your knowledge and teaching opportunities within the yoga fitness industry. YogaFit incorporates the latest scientific research to ensure that safe and effective practices are taught. For more information on any of the teacher training programs or partnering and franchise opportunities included in this appendix, please visit www.yogafit.com.

## YogaFit's Teacher Training Program

YogaFit, the company, and its teacher training program, have expanded considerably since the first training in 1994. YogaFit now features internationally renowned certification programs for yoga and fitness professionals. YogaFit has trained over 200,000 yoga professionals at facilities in the United States and internationally, and it has been integral in the practice of yoga becoming a primary part of health club, gym, and spa programs throughout the world.

YogaFit offers over 40 different educational trainings and a broad spectrum of specialty programs, so you can choose how deep you want to delve. YogaFit offers 200- and 500-hour training tracks as well as opportunities to study in depth on subjects of interest such as our 100-hour Yoga for Athletes specialty certification and YogaFit for Warriors, a 100-hour trauma-sensitive specialty certification originally developed to help the U.S. military heal the wounds of war. YogaFit also offers an in-depth yoga therapy program for those interested in sharing the holistic healing aspects of yoga with clients.

Many people come to YogaFit teacher trainings with the intention of deepening their own practice and not to teach yoga. YogaFit welcomes anyone to explore the diverse aspects of the discipline of yoga from an open, objective perspective that focuses on holistic (mind–body) health benefits through YogaFit. YogaFit runs 10 Mind–Body Fitness Conferences (MBFs) per year nationwide. These conferences offer all levels of training in addition to specialty programming. A fun, interactive way to learn, MBFs offer speakers, raffles, gift bags, kirtan (singing chants), and group bonding. YogaFit has corporate offices in Torrance (California), Toronto, and New York. YogaFit partner studios and YogaFit franchise studios exist across the world. YogaFit continues to expand the horizons of yoga and fitness professionals and enthusiasts around the globe.

Taught by YogaFit-trained instructors with in-depth experience and skills in both yoga and fitness, the YogaFit method is a nationally recognized continuing education credit (CEC) provider for the American Council on Exercise (ACE). It has been a member of the International Health, Racquet and Sportsclub Association (IHRSA) since 1997 and the International Association of Yoga Therapists since 2008. YogaFit is the only yoga instruction certified by Town Sports International (TSI) and New York, Washington, Boston, and Philadelphia Fitness Clubs. YogaFit currently has 60 trainers internationally.

The YogaFit teacher trainings are typically 1 to 4 days of high-quality, hands-on instruction and team teaching. The program provides enough support material to allow you to start teaching your first class right away with confidence. Training classes are held in many locations throughout the United States, Canada, and other countries.

## Community Service Mission and Conscious Business Paradigm

YogaFit is dedicated to community service through community outreach programs from their corporate headquarters and partner studios. We believe that if everyone in the world gave 1 hour per week of community service work, the world would be a better place. This is why we require every YogaFit Level 1 trainee to perform 8 hours of practice teaching in a community service setting before receiving a Certificate of Completion. Our trainees have brought the practice and benefits of yoga to seniors in long-term care homes, stressed-out corporate executives, cancer patients and survivors, people who are terminally ill, children, and the United States military, just to name a few.

The Community Service Program gives our trainees the opportunity to practice their new teaching skills in a less stressful environment with an appreciative audience. As the thousands of letters we receive in our corporate office declare, volunteering time and energy has proven to be the most rewarding experience for many of our trainees. YogaFit is dedicated to this work because it promotes the essence of giving and sharing freely.

YogaFit is a green company and encourages green business practices. YogaFit also encourages and supports the philosophy of conscious business. In this millennium we believe the companies that are socially responsible will prosper from good will and good karma. Together we are changing the paradigm of what it means to do good business—really *good* business.

## YogaFit Studio Franchise

You can now own your own YogaFit studio through our franchise opportunity. The sleek design of the YogaFit studios presents a bright and inviting environment that your students will love to return to day after day. Business is made simple with the proven turnkey systems, financing options, and world-class support. You will be working with a team of seasoned professionals who understand what it takes to make a difference for you and your business.

# YogaFit Partner Program

Are you trained in YogaFit and want to call your classes YogaFit? Then the YogaFit Partner Program is for you. This program allows either a club or studio owner employing YogaFit-trained instructors, or individual YogaFit-trained instructors themselves, to partner with YogaFit and use the powerful YogaFit brand name in marketing your services (only applies to accounts within the United States). Just send us your name, facility, phone, fax number, and e-mail, and we'll get back to you with details. We look forward to working with you and having you join the YogaFit team of partners.

## YogaFit Club Series (YCS)

The YogaFit Club Series offers prechoreographed workouts for health clubs and spas to take the guesswork and liability out of their yoga classes. YCS offers DVDs, CDs, and workout formats to participating clubs and instructors.

## Yoga Alliance

Through YogaFit's comprehensive 200- and 500-hour teacher training programs, you can become a registered yoga teacher (RYT) with the Yoga Alliance, a nonprofit organization that supports yoga teachers and upholds the diversity and integrity of yoga. This certification gives you the professional credibility and experience now sought by health clubs and studios.

## American Council on Exercise (ACE)

YogaFit has chosen the American Council on Exercise (ACE) as its premier provider of fitness certifications. ACE is the only certifying body to offer four fitness certifications accredited by the National Commission for Certifying Agencies (NCCA): group exercise instructor, personal trainer, lifestyle weight management, and clinical exercise specialist.

## Medical Fitness Network

YogaFit is proud to announce our partnership with the Medical Fitness Network in 2015. This network reaches clients with chronic medical conditions who are looking for yoga professionals to help in the day-to-day management of their condition. YogaFit is the exclusive Therapeutic Yoga Program Partner of the Medical Fitness Network.

At YogaFit we believe that therapeutic yoga can positively impact those affected with serious ailments. The Medical Fitness Network (MFN) is a volunteer-driven organization, providing a free, national fitness and health care referral service to those with (chronic) medical conditions—and everyone else! For more information, please visit www.medicalfitnessnetwork.org.

# Yogic Diet and Nutrition

The foundation of any yoga and fitness practice is a healthy diet that provides nourishment to your body to carry you through your day and through your yoga practice. Without vital nutrients, your body becomes weak and leaves a door open for illness and disease.

**Your body looks like what you put into it.**

The purpose of eating is to supply energy to create a healthy, strong, and flexible body. Your body supports you in everything you do. You are what you eat! When you eat, you supply your being with not only calories for energy production but also the life-force energy called prana (also called *chi*). Foods high in sugar, chemicals, pesticides, and other additives are devoid of prana and deplete your body of energy. Besides nourishing your body, prana also clears your mind and boosts your spirit. You know from experience that when you eat well, you feel better on all levels. That's the power of prana. The best nutritional program for those serious about their yoga practice involves simple, fresh, clean, and natural foods.

**Can YogaFit help you lose weight if you need to? Absolutely. If you are truly in touch with your body, you will not overindulge or eat unhealthy foods. The more you practice YogaFit, the more awareness you will build and the more you will notice how various foods affect your body and your mind. A YogaFit workout not only makes you sweat, burn calories, and increase your metabolism, yoga can help shed pounds through addressing mental and emotional issues. Understanding *why* you eat is just as important as regulating *what* you eat and *when* you eat. The result is a healthier body, mind, and spirit. Take time in your mountain III poses to practice awareness—not just how you feel, but what you feel and why. Off your mat, use this same awareness to decide what your body really needs and when.**

Each day, you make important decisions on what to put into your body. Your diet choices either benefit or harm your health. When your daily choices become a lifelong pattern, the beneficial or detrimental consequences can be significant.

# What Is a Yogic Diet?

If you visit places in India, such as the village of Rishikesh (the birthplace of yoga), it is easy to follow the traditional yogic diet, which is vegetarian. Alcohol is also absent from the Rishikesh diet, and so is much of the processed foods found in U.S. supermarkets (and throughout the world, including India). Villagers make their meal choices with the health of their bodies and their spirits in mind. The diet includes an abundance of fresh vegetables, fruits, whole grains, legumes, and fresh milk, likely from the family cow.

The traditional diet of yogis as well as of Hinduism and Buddhism (two major religions in India) is vegetarian, and it reflects the yogic philosophy of yamas and niyamas as discussed in chapter 1. The first yama, ahimsa, is nonviolence to yourself and all living creatures; many yogis choose to become vegetarian to practice ahimsa. Shaucha (purity) is seen in the diet as well. Yogis strive to choose foods that are pure and nonprocessed. Yogis believe that the diet should nourish the body with foods containing prana, such as pure fruits, grains, and vegetables, while avoiding foods that overstimulate the digestive system. This approach to nutrition is called *sattvic* (meaning "real" or "pure") and involves choosing a diet that's wholesome and pure to promote good health, lightness, and higher consciousness.

The Academy of Nutrition and Dietetics acknowledges what traditional yogis have known for centuries. "Many people make the switch to a vegetarian diet because of the potential health benefits. According to the 2010 Dietary Guidelines, vegetarian eating patterns have been associated with improved health outcomes including lower levels of obesity, a reduced risk of heart disease and lower blood pressure. Also, vegetarians tend to consume a lower proportion of calories from fat and fewer overall calories, and more fiber, potassium and vitamin C than non-vegetarians. These characteristics, plus lifestyle factors, may contribute to the health benefits among vegetarians" (AND 2015). Other reasons for choosing a vegetarian diet include a concern for the environment and personal taste preferences. The website for the Academy of Nutrition and Dietetics (www.eatright.org) presents several articles about vegetarianism and the different types.

# Do Yogis Have to Be Vegetarians?

Many Westerners begin yoga with no interest in adopting a vegetarian lifestyle, and that is all right. If that's the case with you, there remain many ways for you to alter your current diet to increase your health and take inches off your waistline if needed, and they are friendly toward the environment. Making small changes can create positive shifts in health and weight management. Eating a diet higher in fruits, vegetables, whole grains, nuts, and fish is associated with lower incidence of heart disease, diabetes, high blood pressure, and other lifestyle-related diseases. The greater dietary changes that are made, the greater the positive health shifts can be. Following are some suggestions to begin to shift toward a yogic diet.

- Go meatless once a week or more. Substitute meat protein with legumes, nuts, lean cheese or other lean dairy, and eggs.

- Make the focus of your meal the vegetables and the meat the condiment.

- If you do eat meat, make a conscious effort to eat meat that is humanely raised and slaughtered and, in the case of fish, is sustainably caught.

- Make your plate colorful by choosing various vegetables each meal.

- Emphasize unrefined carbohydrates, such as vegetables, fruits, whole grains, legumes, nuts, and seeds. These foods are high in fiber, which is beneficial for both health and weight loss.

- Avoid saturated, partially hydrogenated, and trans fats. Saturated fats are mostly found in animal products. Partially hydrogenated fats are found in margarines, many processed foods, baked goods, and snack foods.

- Include foods rich in omega-3 fatty acids, such as cold-water fish (salmon, mackerel, cod), walnuts, macadamia nuts, canola oil, flax seed, kale, and dark, leafy greens. Omega-3 fatty acids reduce inflammation, lower triglycerides, lower blood pressure, and are good for brain health. (In the case of congestive heart failure and chronic angina, avoid omega-3 fatty acids.)

- Choose non-GMO foods.

- Choose foods that are locally produced whenever possible.

- Avoid fried foods.

- Drink plenty of water.

- Avoid sodas and diet sodas.

- Shop the perimeter of the grocery store where the fresh food is kept.

- Consider getting tested to see if you are gluten intolerant.

- If it is *made* in a plant, eat less of it; if it *comes* from a plant, eat more of it.

- Pay attention to how various foods make you feel, and choose foods that give you energy and a feeling of lightness.

Every day offers you an opportunity to make healthy choices; good health is simply a result of making positive choices on a regular basis. The good news is you get to choose—exercise over being sedentary, water over soda, fresh over fried, and supplements over sugar. Experts say it takes 21 days to form a good habit. The nutritional strategies presented here, combined with a regular yoga practice, adequate rest, and time out for meditation and relaxation, can have a dramatic impact on your health and well-being. Healthy habits regarding nutrition might also move you to make more dramatic changes to your diet and lifestyle, such as becoming a vegetarian. However, if you feel overwhelmed at the thought of making major changes overnight, keep in mind that yoga is meant to be a process. Every change, no matter how small, can make a difference. Take one step at a time, listen to your body, and the rewards you receive will be enough to inspire you to keep moving forward on your journey to a stronger and healthier mind, body, and spirit.

Academy of Nutrition and Dietetics. 2015. Vegetarianism: The basic facts. www.eatright .org/resource/food/nutrition/vegetarian-and-special-diets/vegetarianism-the-basic-facts

Bhavanani, A.B., Sanjay, Z., Madanmohan. 2011. Immediate effect of sukha pranayama on cardiovascular variables in patients of hypertension. *International Journal of Yoga Therapy,* 21: 73-76.

Carlson, L.E., Beattie, T.L., Giese-Davis, J., Faris, P., Tamagawa, R., Fick, L.J., Degelman, E.S., and Speca, M. 2015. Mindfulness-based cancer recovery and supportive-expressive therapy maintain telomere length relative to controls in distressed breast cancer survivors. *Cancer,* 121: 476-484. doi: 10.1002/cncr.29063

Epel, E.S., Lin, J., Wilhelm, F.H., Wolkowitz, O.M., Cawthon, R., Adler, N.E., Dolbier, C., Mendes, W.B., Blackburn E.H. 2006. Cell aging in relation to stress arousal and cardiovascular disease risk factors. *Psychoneuroendocrinology,* 31(3): 277-287.

Gothe, N., Pontefex, M.B., Hillman, C., McAuley, E.. 2013. The acute effects of yoga on executive function. *Journal of Physical Activity & Health,* 10(4): 488-95.

Lavretsky, H., Epel, E.S., Siddarth, P., Nazarian, N., Cyr, N. St., Khalsa, D.S., Lin, J., Blackburn, E. and Irwin, M.R. 2013. A pilot study of yogic meditation for family dementia caregivers with depressive symptoms: effects on mental health, cognition, and telomerase activity. *Int. J. Geriat. Psychiatry,* 28: 57–65. doi: 10.1002/gps.3790.

Satchidananda, S.S. 1990. *The Yoga Sutras of Patanjali.* Yogaville, VA: Integral Yoga Publications.

Streeter, C.C., Whitfield, T.H., Owen, L., Arch, B., Rein, T., Karri, S.K., Yakhkind, A., Perlmutter, R., Prescot, A., Renshaw, P.F., Ciraulo, D.A., and Jensen, J.E. 2010. Effects of yoga versus walking on mood, anxiety, and brain GABA levels: A randomized controlled MRS study. *J Altern Complement Med.* Nov; 16(11): 1145-1152. doi: 10.1089/acm.2010.0007. PMCID: PMC3111147

Tolle, Eckhart. 2004. *The power of now.* Vancouver, BC: Namaste.

Villemure, C., Čeko, M., Cotton, V.A., Bushnell, C. 2013. Insular cortex mediates increased pain tolerance in yoga practitioners. *Cerebral Cortex.* http://newsroom. ucla.edu/portal/ucla/how-to-build-a-bigger-brain-91273.aspx.

| Pose name | Page number | Mountain I | Valley I | Mountain II | Valley II | Mountain III |
|---|---|---|---|---|---|---|
| Ab Work | 56 | X | | X | | X |
| Airplane | 126 | X | | X | | |
| Balancing Half Moon | 102 | | | X | X | |
| Big Toe Hold | 212 | | | | | X |
| Big-Toe Wide Boat | 62 | | | | | X |
| Bird of Paradise | 114 | | | X | X | |
| Boat | 60 | | | | | X |
| Bound Side Angle and Bound Triangle | 92 | | | X | | |
| Bow and Half Bow | 152 | | | | | X |
| Bridge | 154 | X | | | | X |
| Bridge on a Block | 309 | X | | | | X |
| Butterfly | 200 | | | | | X |
| Camel | 148 | | | | | X |
| Cat and Cow | 142 | X | | X | | X |
| Chair and Balance Chair | 94 | X | X | X | | |
| Child's Pose | 184 | X | | X | | X |
| Cobra | 46 | X | X | X | | X |
| Crocodile and Kneeling Crocodile | 44 | X | X | X | | |
| Crow | 64 | | | X | | X |
| Dancer | 110 | | | | X | |
| Dead Bug | 210 | | | | | X |
| Dolphin | 124 | | | X | | X |
| Downward-Facing Dog | 122 | X | | X | | X |
| Downward-Facing Dog on the Wall | 302 | X | | X | | X |
| Downward-Facing Dog With Egg Blocks | 303 | X | | X | | X |
| Eagle | 106 | | | | X | |
| Elephant Pose and Eight-Angle Pose | 66 | | | | | X |
| Final Relaxation | 228 | | | | | X |
| Fish | 220 | | | | | X |
| Forward Splits | 190 | | | | | X |
| Frog | 198 | | | | | X |

> continued

> *continued*

| Pose name | Page number | Mountain I | Valley I | Mountain II | Valley II | Mountain III |
|---|---|---|---|---|---|---|
| Side Plank and Kneeling Side Plank | 54 | | | X | | X |
| Spinal Balance | 58 | X | | X | | X |
| Standing Backbend | 144 | | | X | | |
| Standing Balance Pigeon | 108 | | | | X | |
| Standing Big Toe Hold | 112 | | | | X | |
| Standing Chest Expansion With Forward Fold | 130 | X | | X | | X |
| Standing Forward Fold | 120 | X | | X | | |
| Standing Lateral Flexion | 80 | X | | X | | |
| Standing Spinal Twist | 170 | | | | X | |
| Standing Splits | 100 | | | X | X | |
| Standing Straddle Splits | 136 | | | X | | |
| Sun Pose | 78 | X | | X | | |
| Sunbird | 146 | | | X | | X |
| Sunflowers | 76 | X | | | | |
| Supine Half Lotus | 206 | | | | | X |
| Supine Spinal Twist | 178 | | | | | X |
| Supported Cobra, Sphinx, and Locust | 305 | | | | | X |
| Tabletop | 52 | | | | | X |
| Tree | 104 | | | | X | |
| Triangle and Extended Triangle | 88 | | | X | | |
| Triangle With Hand on Thigh or Shin | 301 | | | X | | |
| Turkish Twist | 176 | | | | | X |
| Turtle | 202 | | | | | X |
| Twisting Chair | 166 | | | X | | |
| Twisting Chair—Gentle | 304 | | | X | | |
| Twisting Lunge and Prayer Twisting Lunge | 162 | | | X | | |
| Twisting Triangle | 164 | | | X | | |
| Upside-Down Pigeon | 204 | | | | | X |
| Upward-Facing Dog | 48 | | X | X | | |
| Warrior I | 82 | | | X | | |
| Warrior II | 84 | | | X | | |
| Warrior III | 98 | | | X | X | |
| Wheel | 156 | | | | | X |

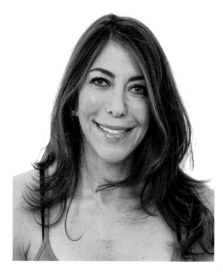

**Beth Shaw** is the president and founder of YogaFit, Inc., the largest yoga school in the world. She is recognized as one of the leading experts in the fields of mind–body fitness, health, and nutrition. Shaw is the innovator behind many fitness trends, including YogaFit, YogaLean, and YogaButt. The first and second editions of *Beth Shaw's YogaFit* (Human Kinetics) have sold more than 100,000 copies worldwide. *YogaLean* was published by Ballantine Books/Random House in 2014 and is quickly climbing to best-seller status. Her next book, *Yoga for Athletes,* is scheduled for release in 2016.

Shaw and her company have been featured in *Time, Huffington Post, USA Today, O: The Oprah Magazine, Glamour, Washington Post, Self, More,* and *Entrepreneur* as well as on CNN, CBS, NBC, Showtime, and E! Entertainment Television. She speaks frequently at universities and corporations on mindfulness in the workplace, health, fitness, and the business of spirituality. Shaw works with the NFL and its officials and is currently on the CanFitPro advisory panel and the Long Island University board of advisors.

Shaw earned bachelor's degrees in business administration and nutrition and holds numerous certificates in fitness disciplines. She is an experienced registered yoga teacher (E-RYT) and is a trained yoga therapist through the International Association of Yoga Therapists (IAYT). She has studied yoga in India and Asia.

A lifelong student of fitness, psychology, philosophy, spirituality, and health, Shaw is committed to helping people find their own perfect health both physically and mentally. YogaFit has committed to giving $1 million in free yoga trainings to those in need. Her nonprofit organization, Visionary Women in Fitness, grants scholarships to women. Shaw has dedicated her life to YogaFit and the transformational growth that the company creates globally. She lives in New York and Los Angeles.